Not No, WAIT

My Painful Journey Through Infertility, Deceit, and Death

Copyright © 2022 by **Angela Sholars King**

All rights reserved. Published by beyondthebookmedia.com

No part of this publication may be reproduced, distributed, or transmitted in any form or by any means, including photocopying, recording, or other electronic or mechanical methods, without the prior written permission of the publisher, except in the case of brief quotations embodied in critical reviews and certain other noncommercial uses permitted by copyright law.

For permission requests, write to the publisher, addressed "Attention: Permissions Coordinator," at the address below. Limit of Liability/Disclaimer of Warranty: While the publisher and author have used their best efforts in preparing this book, they make no representations of warranties with respect to the accuracy or completeness of the contents of this book and specifically disclaim any implied warranties or merchantability or fitness for a particular purpose.

No warranty may be created or extended by sales representatives or written sales materials. The advice and strategies contained herein may not be suitable for your situation. You should consult with a professional where appropriate. Neither the publisher nor author shall be liable for damages arising here from, Beyond The Book Media, LLC. Alpharetta, GA. www.beyondthebookmedia.com

The publisher is not responsible for websites that are not owned by the publisher.

ISBN 978-1-953788-74-0 (Printed)

A NOTE TO THE READERS: Although this book contains the author's personal story, some of the names have been changed for privacy.

Not No, WAIT

My Painful Journey Through Infertility, Deceit, and Death

Angela Sholars King

Dedication

I would like to dedicate *Not No, WAIT* to my daughter, Alexis Renee King. You are the reason for me writing about my journey of deceit and infertility. Every time I look at you, I am reminded of how much Jesus loves me. I thank God for you daily.

I love you, Alexis, and I am so honored to be your mother. My special gift from God. I am so proud of you! Keep letting your light shine!

Always remember, "For **Alexis** can do everything (all things) through Christ, who gives **Alexis** strength." Philippians 4:13 (Personalized and NLT)

In Loving Memory

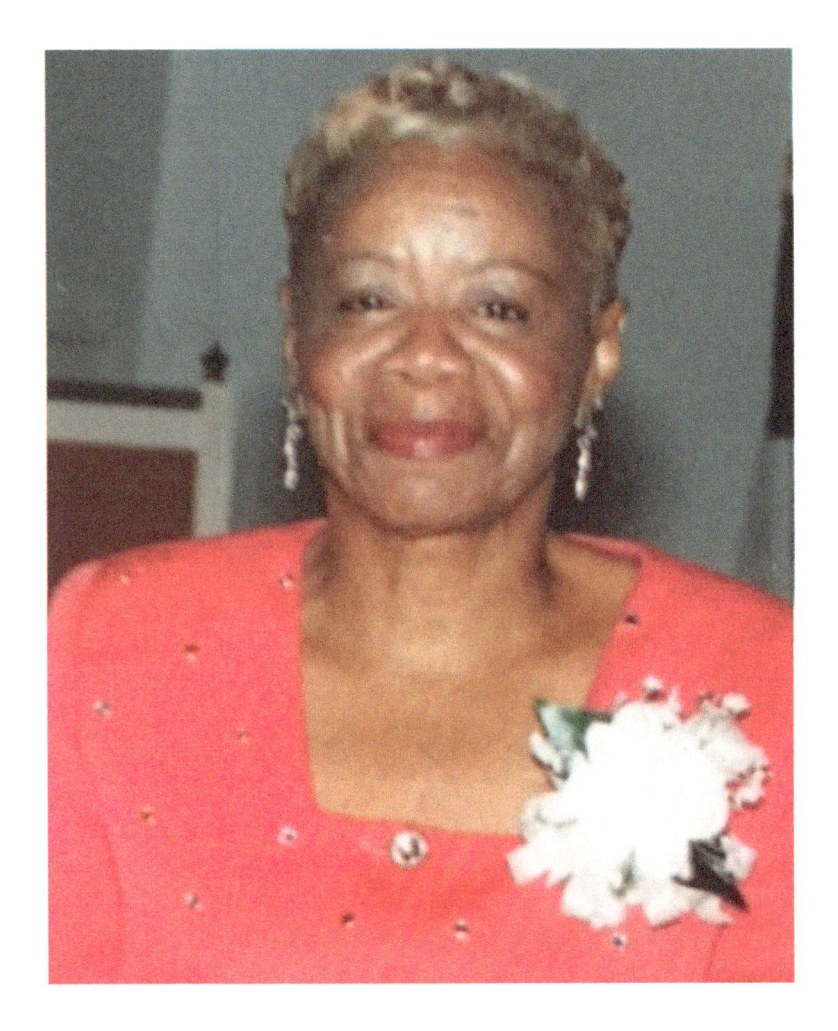

My mother, the late Mrs. Willie Mae Crayton Sholars

Table of Contents

Dedication   5
In Loving Memory   7
About the Author   10
Preface   12

Chapter 1
   Where Do I Start?   15

Chapter 2
   Growing Up Too Fast   23

Chapter 3
   What Is This?   29

Chapter 4
   Let Me See   35

Chapter 5
   Okay, I Accept   39

Chapter 6
   I Love My Doctor   43

Chapter 7
   Okay, Mom. I Will Do It   47

Chapter 8
   Now What?   55

Chapter 9
   Married and Still No Child   63

Chapter 10
   Excited - #Two   71

Chapter 11
   Nervous - #Three   83

Chapter 12
   Afraid - #Four   91

Chapter 13
   Broken - #Five   99

Chapter 14
   I Need a Miracle   105

Chapter 15
   My Gift from God   117

Alexis from Conception through 22 years old   125

About the Author

Angela Sholars King is an ordained minister, certified life coach, and life agent. Angela is nationally known in ministry as the Warrior of Intercession, Deliverance, and Spiritual Warfare. Angela is a World Leader who has partnered with many at all levels of state, business professionals, and international leaders. Angela answered the call and has successfully equipped and empowered many to maximize their leadership potential in their communities and transform souls through the power of prayer. As one of the leading voices for such a time as this, she founded: Women Praying for Christ Ministry, Inc. (WPFCM) with chapters in Liberia, Sierra Leone, Kenya, Nigeria, Texas, and North Carolina, Dr. Angela S. King Ministries, Coach ASK, Women Lets Talk, How will I know, the word of God? The Wailing Hour and Powerful D.I.V.A.S. Angela has developed programs and services for individuals and families needing counseling, prayer, and personal improvement. Her accomplishments as an Evangelist, Teacher, Motivational Speaker, Mentor, Talk Show Host, Life Coach, and now Author have established her as one of the nation's most respected and sought-after voices today. Angela is also a life agent with Primerica Financial Services, in which Angela and her husband are Regional Vice Presidents and run a successful financial services business. Angela decided to write this book under the guidance of the Holy Spirit to minister to women worldwide. Remember," **Have faith." "Don't give up**

on God." "Fight for your family." "God loves you and wants the best for you." "What the enemy means for bad, God will always work it out for your good." Angela resides in Texas with her husband and daughter. She recognizes that she can do absolutely nothing without her Lord and Savior. Her life statement is personalized by Philippians 4:13 (KJV): "Angela can do all things through Christ which strengthens Angela!"

Websites

Coach ASK–angelasking.com

Women Praying for Christ, Inc. – wpfcm.org

Preface

I decided to write this small painful portion of my life story. This book focuses on my very private season of infertility, deceit, and death. I didn't realize that I had buried so many of the events deep down in my subconscious. All of the pain resurfaced when I started to write this book. My prayer is that this book will be an instrument to draw people closer to God and lean into His promises. Reading this book will truly show you how much God loves us all. It will also remind you that you must have faith in God and never give up. You will come to realize that you are stronger than you think. I would have never thought that I could have gone through the things I have in my life, been in my right mind, and written a book about it.

This book was also written in dedication to my daughter Alexis. I wanted her to know how loved and special she is. Not only to God but to me as well. She was the desire of my heart, and God blessed me with her because of my faith in Him.

Angela Sholars King

Email: angela@angelasking.com

Social Media
IG: angelarsking
IG: coachask_angela_s_king
IG: womenprayingforchrist
Facebook: Angela Sholars King
Facebook: Coach ASK – Angela S. King
Facebook: Women Praying for Christ Ministries
Facebook: Praying for Christ Worship Center
Twitter: @drangelasking
Twitter: @CoachASKAngela1
Clubhouse: @angelasking

Chapter 1

Where Do I Start?

"Happiness is never something you get from other people. The happiness you feel is in direct proportion to the love you give."
~~Oprah Winfrey

Meet Angela! The oldest of five siblings from Shreveport, Louisiana. We lived on North Market Street in our first home. It was a lovely spacious home with many snakes and lizards in the neighborhood. I learned at an early age that when you chop a snake in half, it would still be alive and moving. I know that is a little graphic! I remember my first encounter with a blue runner snake while playing in the backyard. I turned around to see a snake flying toward me. To say the least, I was in shock. It stopped in mid-air and turned around as soon as my father opened the back door and called my name, Ann. He was the only person who called me Ann. He noticed the snake from the kitchen window and came to my rescue.

I remember a large hill across the street from our home with red clay dirt on it. That clay dirt had something magical that I loved eating. It was delicious! I loved mud pies and mud cakes and pretended they were real cakes and pastries. Paper dolls used to be my guests for the mud feasts; I loved playing with them. Our home had a driveway that was up on a hill. One day, while playing hide-and-seek, I decided to hide in my father's car. As a fantasy of a seven-year-old, I decided to drive the vehicle. I managed to put the car in reverse, and it started to roll backward from the driveway into the street. There was traffic coming down the road. There came my father to the rescue again! He ran behind the car and stopped it just in time from rolling out into the street. My dad was so strong!

It was time to move. We moved to our second home on Looney Street. It was a nice neighborhood. We lived in a home with a large front porch closed in and a large area under our home. I do not precisely remember what it was called, but it was more of a home with a basement. We could only enter it from the backyard from the long steps that led down to that area. I played under the house a lot. It was very spacious with furniture and other items. My dad bought us bunny rabbits, whom I loved to feed. My favorite time of the week was Friday evening when my dad would take me to get a hamburger, fries, and a shake. Those were the best hamburgers I have ever tasted. Believe it or not, I had a speech problem during my early elementary school years. I was shy and always stuttered. But thank the Lord; I grew out of it.

I loved walking to the neighborhood store to purchase candy. Like every child, that was my favorite thing to do, and just like every other child, I hated oatmeal. But my father expected my mother to make it every morning for breakfast, and I was expected to eat it, which I secretly never did. Instead, I used to give my portion to my brother, and if he did not want it, I simply poured it down the washing machine pipe. But all this mischief of mine was soon to be caught.

One day, I was playing under the house when my father called my name. I didn't hear him, and soon he was under the house with me. He asked if I heard him calling my name, and I said, "No, sir." Back then, you always said yes or no, sir or ma'am. The next thing I knew, I was looking past my father at the oatmeal on the ground behind him. The washing machine water drained down under the house, and the oatmeal that I had placed down the pipe was sitting on top of the soil. My father turned around to see what I was looking at, and he discovered my dark secret. Well, you know what happened after that. I was in a lot of trouble.

When I was eight years old, my mother informed us that she was leaving Louisiana. She was going to Texas to find a place for us to live. *"I will return to get you, and then we will live in Texas,"* she said. I did not understand what was happening at all. We remained with my father, and my mother left for Texas with my baby brother. It was not long before my father convinced my mother to return to LA, and she did. Little did I know that my father was unfaithful and abusive to my mother. He was very smart with his actions when it concerned me; he never let us see or hear the abuse. Well, or so I thought.

I discovered later in life that he was using me to see his mistress on Fridays when he took me for hamburgers. I used to see the lady and always wondered how she knew my name and seemed to know a lot about me. My father continued with his immoral behavior, according to my mother, after she returned to try to make the marriage work. After having enough, my mother decided to leave my father again. This time she took all of us with her to Texas. Of course, it is never a pleasing experience for a child to see his or her parents separating. As a child, I thought it would not be that hard for me, but life is not always what it seems.

No one should underestimate how traumatic and disturbing separation can turn out for the children. After moving to Texas, we lived with one of our aunts for some time while mom looked for work and a place for us to live. Soon, my mom started her life as a working woman. She was a lady who had never worked in her entire life, but life turned out different for her after the separation. Thus, being a mom of four children at that time, she had to work day and night to take care of us.

It did not take her very long before she had enough money to move into our own apartment. This was quite different for us. We had never lived in an apartment before. Later, we discovered it was a low-income area, and the apartments we lived in were considered "the projects." Everyone was nice and friendly in that neighborhood. Soon, my siblings and I enrolled in school and started living a normal day-to-day life. I witnessed my first fight between two girls on my way home from school; that was something I had never seen before. My teachers at school were really caring about every child, and I loved them all.

Things were extremely hard for my mom. She worked two and three jobs to provide us with all the necessary things in life. I will never forget that my mom tried her best for us. Even when she was tired, even when she was worried, strained, and stressed, she did it all for us. She had every intention of being good, grand, and great, but it was just too hard for her some days. Luckily, she was blessed to have two sisters and one brother in Texas.

Since I was the oldest daughter and firstborn, dad and I were close. He was the first man I ever loved and the first hand I ever held. During the summers, I was overly excited because it was when we traveled back and forth from Texas to Louisiana to visit him. It was one of my favorite times since I missed him very much. But this happiness would soon change.

After my parents separated, I realized what responsibilities really are. At the tender age of eight, I was expected to keep things in order since I was the oldest. I took care of my siblings while my mom worked. At that time, I did not pay much attention to this, but now I realize it was a lot of responsibility to place on a child's shoulder. It's good to have discipline in the household, but each child must get to live their childhood fully. That's what childhood is all about.

After some time, my mom conceived my sister, and we were now five children: three boys and two girls. I was now ten years old. Within a year or two after the birth of my sister, my mom moved us into a home. She never re-married, nor did my father. In fact, they never divorced. My mother was a religious woman and sang in the church choir. She had a beautiful voice. Her words would sound like the angels praising God in the listener's ears. She was a kind woman and spent all her energy raising us well. As they say, *"A beautiful woman uses her lips for truth, her voice for kindness, her ears for compassion, her hands for charity, and her heart for love. For those who do not like her, she uses prayer."*

I would say this is the perfect definition of what my mother looked like. She did not play around and always taught us to be kind to ourselves and others. My mom inculcated feelings of empathy, compassion, and kindheartedness in me since she always reminded us never to look down upon others. Indeed, I kept the lessons provided by her close to my heart. Maybe as a child, I did not take them seriously or did not understand them well, but now I perfectly understand how well she raised us.

I remember what she always said, *"It's nice to be nice!"* Always reminded us to look into the eyes of people while talking to them and use our words wisely. In fact, we learned more from what she was than from what she taught. Because at the end of the day, the most awe-inspiring key to our development was her positive involvement with us. No matter what, she never left us behind and nurtured us physically, emotionally, and into good humans.

My younger brother passed away when I was in senior high school due to bone cancer. I was devastated. It was shocking for all of us. It was the saddest day of my life, and I wanted to break down; I loved him dearly. But somehow, God gave me the strength to hold it together for myself, my mom, and my siblings. My mother was heartbroken about my brother's death;

he was only fifteen years old. No mother expects to bury their children; I am sure that was a deep hurt she never got over. I remember the hurt that she later shared with me because, at the time, she could not afford to purchase a headstone for my brother's grave. That really crushed her spirit. I watched her go into depression for a short span of time, but she was a fighter. My mom soon fought her way out of it and returned to caring for us. She always used to say, *"Bernie* (that was my brother's nickname) *would not want me to be sad and crying all the time."*

We were now two brothers and two sisters. At that time, being the oldest, I had to help support my mom by taking care of my siblings; there was no room for mistakes or sadness. They all looked up to me. I loved and still love them with all of my heart and soul. My mom always encouraged us to stay close together.

I have always had a nurturing relationship and always wanted the best for each of them. When you hurt one of them, you hurt me as well. There is nothing that I would not do for my siblings. My love for them is unbreakable. They are all successful individuals, and I am extremely proud of them. They have blessed me with wonderful nieces, nephews, great-nieces, and great-nephew. I love my siblings from the core of my heart, and they all are still utterly dear to me. I was and will always be very protective of them. As quoted by Michael J. Fox,

"Family is not an important thing. It's everything."

Chapter 2

Growing Up Too Fast

"When we are children, we seldom think of the future. This innocence leaves us free to enjoy ourselves as few adults can. The day we fret about the future is the day we leave our childhood behind."
~~ Patrick Rothfuss

My teenage years flew by, babysitting my siblings. I had to take care of them. But during my childminding, I did not get enough time for myself because I had devoted my childhood to looking after my siblings. Sometimes, I just wanted to be a teenager with no responsibilities and have fun just like other kids my age. I was cleaning and cooking most of the time while my mother worked. Watching my siblings was a daily chore.

Along with the guardianship of my siblings, I also started to work at an incredibly early age (in my teenage years) to help my mom. I worked as a secretary at the local community center.

My experience as a teenager in middle and high school was good. I had my group of friends, and we were remarkably close. My main goal was to remain active in school always, both academically and socially. The most fun part of school was when I spent time with my friends. I remember the exciting times at lunch, football games, track, booster club, Allied Youth, Distributive Education Clubs of America, Flag Girl, Pep Rallies, and parties.

I grew up to be a surprisingly good young lady. Along with taking care of my siblings, I also tried to take time for myself. As high school days came closer, life became even more fun. I was chosen as Valentine's Sweetheart in high school. But still, I did not have much time for dating. My top priority was to finish school and take care of my siblings.

> *"With self-discipline most anything is possible."*
> *~~ Theodore Roosevelt*

After some time, I started tutoring young students to make some extra money. I felt like it was probably the most effective way to keep my learning process active. I was a student and believed that the more you teach others about a certain idea or subject, the more you learn. I started to teach two students who were brother and sister. I used to walk to their home to tutor them. They needed my help in English, History, and Math, and I was more than happy to take on this job.

I would tutor them after school. Since it got pretty dark by the time I returned home, sometimes my brothers would meet me at the park and walk with me back home. But obviously, this was not a daily routine, and I had to look after myself while returning home on several occasions during the night. No doubt, it was terrifying. I saw boys doing drugs in the park, and there were needles on the ground. Although no one ever bothered me, a ripple of fear used to run down my spine whenever I saw them.

At the end of the week, the most awaited time was when I got my paycheck. It made me feel confident in myself. I felt glad that I could help my mother and reduce the financial burden on her shoulders. On my payday, I would buy small things for my siblings that made them happy. Seeing them happy made me feel happy. I learned at an early age that it was a good feeling to have your own money.

I graduated high school at 17 years old. As a matter of fact, I was blessed to graduate high school early because I started first grade at five years old. All of my family members and friends attended my graduation ceremony. It was one of the most memorable days of my life. I felt delighted and proud, but I also had a feeling of fear deep within myself, as if everything was about to change in my life. I was bound to a dozen conflicting emotions, but the primary feeling was a sense of pride. Graduating high school was a big deal, and I felt delighted to walk across that stage and get my diploma.

After graduation, I enrolled in college and moved into my own apartment. This was when I decided to start dating as I had grown up. I was looking forward to having this time, but despite the sentimental feelings, I wanted to take some precautions. I had seen my mom go through so much and did not want to experience the same things, or maybe you could say that the circumstances in my life had made me a little sensible at an early age.

Thus, I decided to take some precautionary actions before I started dating. I went to Planned Parenthood because I had thought of using birth control. I was not sure if it was a good idea, but there was no harm in getting a consultant there and starting to use it. Therefore, I did not tell anyone about my idea and went there alone. I knew for a fact that I didn't want to get pregnant out of wedlock or have children before marriage. It was something I always wanted to stay away from. After watching my mother struggle so much with us, I never wanted to go through that type of life. I didn't want that for myself or my children.

It was a sunny afternoon when I walked across the rigid black-crown sidewalk of the Planned Parenthood building and entered. I had already scheduled an appointment and waited for the doctor for some time. Keeping my feet flat on the floor, my hands rolled around one another close to my chest, and I waited for the receptionist to call out my name.

Soon enough, I found myself in the doctor's room, where he examined me. I had not imagined the examination to be as stressful and painful as it was. I will never forget the discomfort I felt in that room. The instrument that the doctor used was extremely painful. Leaning back on the examination bed, I thought to myself, *what in the world are they about to do to me?*

A sigh of relief left my lips as the doctor told me the examination was over. In the back of my mind, I thought the trouble was over, and now I would be handed over a paper with the name of the birth control pills written on it, but things were about to take a tragic turn.

After the examination, the doctor turned around and told me that I had fibroid tumors which were located on the walls of my uterus. I had no idea what fibroid tumors were or what he meant by that. I was unable to judge anything since the way he said it seemed like it was a very normal thing and could be cured by medicine. For instance, I did not feel worried until I raised an eyebrow and requested him to explain in common terms what that meant exactly.

"This means that you can never have children," he said. After dropping this news in my lap, the doctor showed no emotions. Right then, I felt devastated and knew my life was about to change.

In a state of terror and shock, I left the room. For a moment, I felt like everything around me had gone dark. I was not ready for that news, nor did I know what to feel in such a situation. I was a perfectly fine woman having no mental or physical health problems. I always had been healthy and never showed any symptoms, pain, or discomfort. Sitting in the hallway for a moment to digest what I had just heard, I walked out of the building, thinking I needed to call my mom right now.

I needed to tell my mom everything and get myself checked for a second opinion. Part of me did not believe this at all. The other part of me said, *"You need to find out if this is, in fact, really true."* I knew that Planned Parenthood was a place for low-income and uninsured individuals, and so I questioned the news the doctor had given to me. In fact, I always questioned the information I received from them and whether they had my best interest in mind.

> **"And the child grew and became strong, filled with wisdom. And the favor of God was upon him."**
> ~~**Luke 2:40 (ESV)**

Chapter 3

What Is This?

"My mama always said, life is like a box of chocolates. You never know what you're gonna get."
~~Forrest Gump

I stopped by my mom's house to tell her the bad news. I could hardly get the words out of my mouth, let alone in the right order. I could not breathe. My head started to hurt really bad. My mom asked me to calm down and speak slowly.

I explained to my mom what the doctor told me at Planned Parenthood. My mother became very upset with me. She asked me why I would go to planned parenthood in the first place. I explained to her my reasoning, and I wanted to do it myself. My mother was unhappy and did not believe the information that the doctor gave to me. She decided to make an appointment for me with her gynecologist.

My appointment was not for three days from the day that I received the bad news. I thought that I would go crazy before that day came. I was nervous and needed to know the truth. Those three days seemed like three years. It seemed to go by so slowly.

The day has finally arrived! It's the day of my doctor's appointment. My mother went with me to my appointment. Doctor K. did a few tests, examined me, and confirmed that there were four fibroid tumors in the wall of my uterus. The tears could not stop running down my face. I really lost it.

He explained the whole thing to me, telling me they could get larger and increase in number. I was devastated, and I cried for days. To this day, no one has an answer for where these fibroid tumors come from. I continued to ask him questions. How and why did this happen to me? What are these, and where do they come from? Are you sure there is nothing that I could take to get rid of them? Are they cancerous? Can you shrink them? Why do I have these when no one else in my family has these? Are you sure of your findings?

I had questions upon questions until I could not think of anything else to ask. Doctor K. was a very patient man. He took his time and answered each of my questions to the best of his ability. He really spent a lot of time with me. I know he had other patients waiting. However, he never rushed me or made me feel he didn't care. I felt he was the best doctor in the world at that moment. The next statement that came out of his mouth stopped my heart from beating for a few seconds. Doctor K. informed me that I would probably never be able to have children due to the location of the fibroids. I asked him to leave the room and give me a minute to process all this information. He said he would check back with me in about 15 minutes.

My mother tried her best to comfort me. At that time, I could not be comforted. My emotions were all over the place. I was numb. *This cannot be real. Surely, I am dreaming and having a nightmare.* Now my head was killing me, and my eyes were red. I was not in the best mental state. *I just want to go to sleep. When I wake up, this will all be a bad dream.* Well, reality hit me in the chest. I am awake, and this is all real.

Doctor K. comes back into the room. He asked me how I was handling all of this info. Of course, I informed him that I was not doing well at all. He asked me if I had any additional questions, and I said no. He informed me that he would like to schedule me for a six-month follow-up appointment. This would be to check and see if the fibroids have gotten any larger. He also asked me to call his office if I started feeling pain or discomfort. He reassured me that I would be fine and to take it one day at a time.

I left his office. My mother was driving, and I was still in shock. No conversation took place during this drive home. I didn't want to talk about it at all. My mother stopped to get us something to eat. I really didn't have an appetite at all. I just wanted to get home and go to bed. It seemed like the longest ride home that I had ever had.

After arriving home, I went straight to my room. I didn't want any food or company. I just wanted to be alone and think. Here I am, a first-year college student, and a doctor tells me I will never have children. How am I expected to understand this? I have not done anything in life to deserve this.

Why am I being punished? I can never be a complete woman. I was told that you go to school, get an education, get a good job, get married, and have children. No one prepared me for this type of news. *What is wrong with me? Why was I born different? This is just not fair. I have been robbed of being a mother and probably a wife. What man will want to marry me if he finds out I cannot have children? I have taken good care of my siblings all my life, and now I am told I can never have children. I have been a good child. I never really gave my parents any trouble.* **WHY IS THIS HAPPENING TO ME**? *I just don't understand this.*

I decided to stay home from school the next day. I am still not in the mood to see anyone. I finally started to open up and talk to my mother about it. She reminded me not to look at what I saw. She reminded me that doctors only know so much, but God has the final say. I asked her why God would let this even happen to me. She reminded me that bad things happen to good people. However, it will always work out for my good if I believe.

Believe in what? She reminded me to believe that God can do anything. I told her that I knew that. So why did God let this happen to me? My mother did not like it when I questioned God's decisions. I wanted to hear her answer. Besides, moms have all of the answers…so I thought.

My mother held my hand, looked into my eyes, and said, "God does what he wants to do. He does not have to answer to us. But always know that he loves me so much, and he hurts when I hurt."

I, in turn, said something that I should not have said. "Well, I hope God is in pain right now because I truly am."

My mother replied, "I know you are in a lot of pain right now. But please don't let it cloud your thinking, causing you to disrespect God.

I didn't feel at all that I was disrespecting God. I was simply stating how I was feeling. My mother ended the conversation with these words: "Angela, you are a very special young lady. God will turn this around for your good. I feel this in my spirit."

"Okay, mom. I love you. Thank you for listening to me!"

"The LORD is near to all who call on him, to all who call on him in truth."
~~Psalm 145:18 (ESV)

Chapter 4

Let Me See

*"Sometimes you have to just let
go and see what happens"*
~~Self

I continued attending college. I was trying to move on, but this always stayed at the back of my mind. I always thought about not being able to give birth or have children. Dating was the last thing on my mind. I tried to cope with my problem by staying focused on school and keeping myself very busy.

I realized that my problem had truly taken a toll on me. I didn't want to be in any relationship. If the thought came up in my mind and I tried to date, it didn't turn out very well. Guys would always tell me that I didn't act like I really cared about the relationship at all. They actually had every reason to feel that way. I really didn't care at all. I was hurt, sad and confused…all at the same time.

I went through school in a daze. My cover and protection are about to end. It's time to leave my protection (college) and move into the real world. I was blessed to start my professional career in finance. I am working now, moving into my townhome, and about to start living the good life.

I started to travel on the weekends. I loved meeting new people and trying new things. I also loved to dance. I went to nightclubs every Thursday – Saturday. But, on Sundays, I was always in the church at Sunday School and singing in the choir on the front row during service.

Life is passing me by very fast. I am now in my late twenties. Twenty-seven to be exact. I decided to be in a relationship. It was good but not the person I felt I would ever marry. As the months went by, out of curiosity, I decided I wanted to try getting pregnant. Well, to my surprise, it happened…I became pregnant. I was not serious about the pregnancy or my boyfriend. I just wanted to see if what the doctor said was really true. I was pregnant with the wrong person. I should be so happy, but instead, I was very unhappy. I couldn't believe this. I was pregnant when the doctor said that I could never get pregnant. I am so confused and upset. I truly didn't know what to do or how to feel.

What do I do now? I am not married. I never wanted to have a child before marriage. This is not how my life has been planned in my mind. I have to make a decision and make it soon. I can't bring a child into the world this way. I wanted a child, but not like this. What would people think about me? How would my siblings look at me now? Nothing about this is good for me right now, except that I was pregnant, and I was told that this would never happen in my lifetime.

I did not want a child with this guy. I was scared and confused. I decided to do something that was against my religion and morals. I decided to have an abortion. I was scared about a lot of things. Would I ever be able to get pregnant again if I had an abortion? I decided to take the chance and go through with it.

I went to a clinic to have the procedure. I didn't tell anyone or want my doctor to know. After the procedure, I drove myself home. I felt terrible about what I had done. I cried for days and didn't talk to anyone. I took a week off work to heal and get my mind back into focus.

A week after the abortion, I felt really sick. My mother came over to my home and took me to the doctor. After my examination, I was told that I had the flu. I was given several prescriptions to fill and drove back home. After arriving back home, I attempted to take the prescribed medicine. My mother went upstairs to retrieve something from my bedroom. Suddenly, I couldn't move my body or even talk. I tried moving but fell to the floor with my eyes slowly closing. My mother heard it and ran back down the stairs.

She called an ambulance, and the next thing I knew, I was at the hospital with doctors standing over me talking. After running several tests, my mother was informed that I would need emergency surgery. I was bleeding internally. I found out later after the surgery that I did not have the abortion because I had a tubal pregnancy. I was paralyzed because I was bleeding internally due to my fallopian tube bursting. I had to receive five pints of blood. It was also discovered at that time that I had a rare blood type.

I was in the hospital for a week. During that time, I was in a lot of pain. It hurt so bad when they had me to start walking. I had never felt pain like that before. It was necessary if I wanted to go home within a week. No one really knew why I was in the hospital but my mother. I still did not tell anyone else. The father of my unborn child came to see me in the hospital. I never told him why I was in the hospital, and I surly did not let him know that I had been pregnant and attempted to discontinue the pregnancy.

"You will face many defeats in life, but never let yourself be defeated." ~~Maya Angelou

Chapter 5

Okay, I Accept

"I have learned over the years that when one's mind is made up, this diminishes fear."
~~*Rosa Parks*

I was released from the hospital and started my healing process. My mother came to my home to take care of me for four of my six-week recovery time. During the fifth week, I decided to be hardheaded and drive myself to the store. I didn't realize how many muscles you use while driving. I got out of the car and started to walk into the store. My incision started to hurt really bad. I could hardly walk. All of a sudden, I started bleeding. I fell to the floor in tremendous pain.

One of the store employees came and asked me if I was okay. I told him; no, I was not okay. I asked him to please just help me to my car. I drove myself back home while crying all the way. Luckily, I did not live very far from the store.

I called my doctor to inform him of my current situation. He asked me to take off the bandage and look at the incision. I was so afraid because I thought I had pulled something loose and needed another surgery. Thank God it turned out that I didn't. Now I had to tell my mother what I had done. She was not happy, of course, but she was thankful I was okay.

I begin to look over my life. I felt guilt, hurt, and shame because I attempted to do something that went against my morals and religion. The whole experience taught me that we should not be too quick to judge. We often judge women for wanting to become mothers and making the wrong decisions. We never realize what they might be going through mentally and physically. Although no one except my mother knew what had happened, I was still ashamed because my younger siblings saw me as a role model.

I had to accept the fact that I could not have children. I felt bad, I resented other women who had children and could start a family, but I knew it would not happen for me. I started talking to God all the time. I saw careless moms and told God, "These women were not even good parents, yet I do not have a child."

I felt maybe I was being punished because I did something stupid out of curiosity. The pain continued to mount, taking over my every thought. I thought about children and why this was happening to me every day. Why could I not have children? Why did I have those fibroid tumors? WHY, WHY, WHY???

I knew that I needed to accept it. However, I had so many questions in my mind that had not been answered. It just didn't make any sense to me. *How can I accept something that I just don't understand? I have not been a perfect person. I surly am not a bad person.* **WHY***????????*

Maybe it will just disappear if I don't think about it much. Maybe this is all just a very bad nightmare. God would not let this happen to me. Now that's it. This is not real. Surely this is just a bad dream. I will be able to have children. Okay, stop lying to yourself, Angela. You will not be able to have children. You must stop this foolishness and accept that you will never be a mother. No one will ever call you mom. You will never be a grandma. You will never help plan your daughter's or son's wedding. You will never be invited over to your child's home for dinner. No one will ever say to you, "I love you, Mom!" You will never attend your child's graduations. You will never hold a child in your arms and tell them how much you loved and wanted them. You will never be able to pick them up when they fall and let them know they are okay! You will never be able to teach them about God and how Jesus died for their sins. You will never be able to talk to them about Jesus' love.

Well, at the moment, I really don't feel Jesus loves me anymore. How could he not bless me with the one thing He created me to do? Multiply. I don't feel loved by God at all right now. Every dream I have ever had of being a mother has been stripped away from me. I was not even warned. I was just told **NO CHILDREN FOR YOU, ANGELA**, *and you must deal with it. It's hard to breathe just thinking about my life with this huge void. Would any man really want to marry or love me if they knew I couldn't have children?*

What kind of life would I have, knowing I would feel incomplete without having at least one child? How will family and friends view and treat me? This road is going to be too hard to bare. I have to accept it and just move on with my life. **OKAY, I ACCEPT.**

"Life is what happens when you're busy making other plans." ~~John Lennon

Chapter 6

I Love My Doctor

"Whoever is happy will make others happy too."
~~Anne Frank

Well, time continues to move on. It's time for my yearly check-up. I just love my doctor. He's so patient, kind, and understanding. He checks the size of the fibroids yearly to make sure they are not growing or multiplying. I forget they are inside of me. They never hurt or bothered me at all. If I didn't see them during my sonograms, I would not believe they really exist.

My checkup was good, as usual. No change in size at all. I have these non-cancerous, non-painful tumors inside my uterus, causing me to not have children. This is so insane to me. I'm still really having an extremely tough time wrapping my brain around this entire process. Something is growing inside my body, and nobody knows how it got there or why. And to top it all off, this something never gives me any pain or discomfort. My doctor continues to explain that, as long as I have no pain…I should be fine and don't worry about them. If I start to have any major discomfort, I will have a hysterectomy. I have no other options.

No medicine, no treatment plan, or surgery. Just straight to **NO CHILDREN FOR YOU, ANGELA.**

I leave his office numb as I do each year after my checkup. I take that long drive back to work in my renewal state of continued shock. Even though he is nice, he reminds me year after year that I will never be able to have children. That conversation is starting to really get on my last nerve. I am starting to feel like wanting to have children is only important to me. It doesn't seem like anybody else cares but me.

I'm back at work. Smiling and acting like everything is great. I have a wonderful job, making great money, and living my best life. Well, almost my best life. I arrive to work early and work late. This helps me forget about my problem. My company just loves my work ethic. Nobody knows why I work so hard. Working keeps my mind off the real problem, my infertility. Everyone thinks the reason that I am not settling down is because I'm just not ready. I am also not ready to be a mother. That lie is so far from the truth. I must suffer in silence for now. No one can know how deeply hurt I am inside. I am known as the strong one. I can't let anyone see how much pain I am in daily.

I have so many ways to numb the pain. Let's see…I can go partying, dancing, dating, traveling, wining, and dining. Anything to keep my mind off my internal pain. Besides, I'm still young, and people are not really pressuring me that much. To look at me, I would appear carefree, without a problem in the world. That appearance was so far from the truth.

My girlfriends didn't even know how much pain I carried around inside of me daily. Everybody wanted to be like Angela. Angela had it all together, so they thought. If they only knew how I really felt. Especially my friends who had children. They wanted my life, and I wanted their life. Each day started to get harder and harder for me to bare. I just wanted to wake up from this dream and realize that it has only been a dream and I could really have children one day. My wishful thinking worked for about a year or so. I was finally able to forget all about my problem and just enjoy life!

I started to date a young man who lived in another state. This would enable me to travel more and keep myself busier at the same time. I was enjoying life and placed my problem in the very back portion of my mind. I tried to never think about it. I had finally convinced myself that everything was normal. I had no worries at all. I was okay, and everything about me was great!

"Love is patient, love is kind. It does not envy, it does not boast, it is not proud. It does not dishonor others, it is not self-seeking, it is not easily angered, it keeps no record of wrongs."
~~1 Corinthians 13:4-5 (NIV)

Chapter 7

Okay, Mom. I Will Do It

"It is during our darkest moments that we must focus to see the light."
~~Aristotle

I started attending a new church. I really enjoyed it. I loved my new group of friends. We became like family. Every Sunday after church, we would go out to lunch together to enjoy each other's company.

I remember attending a women's conference at the church. I didn't plan to attend. However, one of my friends talked me into attending. While attending the conference, during the lunch break, a group of ladies gathered in a circle to talk. I walked over to hear what they were talking about. Well, to my surprise, they were talking about infertility problems. This is truly a setup, and I should have never walked over into this conversation. This is my buried secret, and I want it to stay that way. I didn't want to talk to anyone about this. I surely didn't want any of the ladies to know my business.

As the conversation continued, one of the ladies decided to ask me a question. Angela, are you happy with your OBGYN? I am now looking at her with a puzzled look and replied, "Yes, I love my doctor."

"Well, I know you love your doctor, but would you be open to seeing a new doctor?"

I am now confused and wondering why she would continue asking me that question. It was like she knew something about me, and I was trying to figure out how she knew and why she was only asking that question.

With a not so holy look on my face, I decided to answer her back.

"I am fine with my doctor. I see no need for a second doctor."

"Well, Angela, I understand you are happy with your doctor. But I have started to go to this new doctor, who is truly the best doctor ever."

She explained how she was having infertility problems and fibroid tumors. She explained that he was the only doctor who would remove her fibroid tumors, and now she has two children.

I tried to keep my posture, eyes, and body language positive. However, I was so shocked that I became speechless. At that moment, I knew this was a setup by God. No one else could have done this, and I knew that no one else knew about my situation. At that moment, my wall began to fall. I began to talk to the ladies about my infertility struggle and how I knew this was a setup from God. I discovered that she had the same type of fibroid tumors in the same location, on the wall of her uterus.

She asked me again if I would be willing to see another doctor and receive a second opinion. Well, of course, my answer was now yes. She gave me the doctor's name, address, and telephone number. I thanked her for the info, and we continued to talk about her past and current situation. I was listening but still in a state of shock. Why is this happening? Should I really make an appointment to see her doctor? I am so confused and afraid.

I attempted to enjoy the remainder of the conference. I must say that I don't remember much about the conference. My mind was too busy replaying that meeting with her during the lunch break. I don't even remember the other ladies in the group discussion. I only remember her.

After the conclusion of the conference, I went home and called my mother and told her about this connection. I was literally talking myself out of calling this new doctor. My mother convinced me to call the doctor and make an appointment. I didn't call his office right away. It took me two weeks to finally make that call. I called to schedule an appointment. I was surprised to get an appointment within the week. Still trying to talk myself out of going. I thought, well, he must not be that good of a doctor. Why was I able to get in to see him so soon?

Days go by, and now it's time for my appointment. I was so afraid for some reason. I have already been given the worst news of my life. Why was I afraid? There was nothing that he could tell me that would be any worst but cancer. I also had a feeling of betrayal from my current doctor. After all, he has been my doctor for many years and is also my mother's doctor.

My name was called. While walking back to the patient room, I really start to sweat. I am so nervous. The nurse asks me questions and takes my height, weight, etc. She informs me that the doctor will be in to see me soon. After about five minutes, I hear a knock on the door. It was the doctor walking into the room. He smiled, shook my hand, and told me it was very nice to meet me. He asked me if anyone referred me to him and, if so who. I informed him of the connection, and we began talking about why I had come to see him today. After explaining my situation, he informed me that he would like to take a sonogram, so he will be able to take a look at the fibroids for size and location. I agreed to the sonogram.

I was taken back into another room by the nurse to take the sonogram. After the completion of the sonogram, I was informed that the doctor would need a few minutes to review it, and he will come back and talk to me about his findings shortly. I was then taken back to my original room to wait for the doctor to return. After about fifteen minutes, the doctor returned. He placed the images up on a screen for us to review together. This was actually the first time that I truly looked at the tumors. There were four of them. Two are the size of a small lemon, and the other two are the size of a quarter.

He showed me that one of them was laying on top of my bowels. This explained why my bowels were never normal. He then asked me whether I wanted to have children.

I looked at him with tears in my eyes and said, "Yes, more than anything in the world. However, my current doctor informed me that I would never be able to have children."

He asked me again, "Do you want to have children?"
"Yes."
He replied, "I can remove these tumors, and you can have children."
I know that I didn't just hear him say that I could be able to have children.
"Are you sure?"
He said, "Of course, I am sure."

I explained to him that my doctor told me this would be a very risky surgery, and no doctor would attempt to try it because the tumors were in the wall of my uterus.

He informed me that it might be too risky for my current doctor but not for him. He performed this type of surgery all of the time with much success. He also said he wanted me to have a child, just as much as I wanted to have one. Just him saying that made me feel so good and at ease. I really have a totally different opinion about this new doctor now. It was a lot to take in at the moment.

He began to explain to me how the procedure would be done, at what hospital, and the recovery process and timeframe. He then asked me when I would like to schedule the surgery. I was still in shock and confused. It all sounded too good to be true. After all, a doctor I trusted 100% told me for so many years that I could never have a child.

I informed him that I needed a little time to think about it. He informed me that the longer I put it off, the worst it could be.

Does this doctor just want to cut on me for his experimental research, or is he truly sincere?

I said I would let him know soon. I checked out and left his office.

After arriving home, I called my mother to tell her about the appointment. Her response was you should go ahead and have the surgery. I told her that I would have to think about it. Weeks went by, and I still had not made a decision. I had this theory of if something does not hurt you, you should leave it alone and not have unnecessary surgery. I decided to ask my mother if she would meet this new doctor with me and tell me what she thinks after meeting him. She agreed, and I scheduled a second appointment with him. During the appointment, my mother asked most of the questions. I just observed and listened. After all the questions had been answered, my mother informed the doctor that we would talk and get back with him. My mother thanked him for his time, and we exited the building.

During our drive home, my mother told me she felt good about him. She really felt that he had my best interest at heart. She encouraged me again to consider having the surgery. I told her again that I would think about it. She asked me, what is it to really think about? I informed her that this would be my body being cut on and not hers. I would need some time to think and weigh all of my options.

After one week of thinking about it and my mother asking me every day when I was going to schedule the surgery, I finally said, "Okay, Mom, I will do it." I called the doctor's office the next day to schedule the surgery.

The nurse called me back with confirmation of the surgery in eight days. She went over all of the details of the surgery and what needed to take place days before the surgery. I called my mother to tell her I had finally scheduled the surgery. She informed me that she would be there with me from beginning to end. Not to worry, because she had a very good feeling about this doctor and the procedure. She felt God's hand upon this connection, and everything God plans is always for our good!

"For I know the plans I have for you, "declares the Lord, "plans to prosper you and not to harm you, plans to give you hope and a future."

~~Jeremiah 29:11 (NIV)

Chapter 8

Now What?

"Too many of us are not living our dreams because we are living our fears."
~~ Les Brown

Well, it's the day of my surgery. Driving to the hospital was a very quiet time. I really didn't want to talk. My mother understood and remained quiet with me. The closer we got to the hospital, the more nervous I became.

We arrived safely, parked the car, and walked into the hospital. I checked in and waited to be called back. The call back came very quickly. It seemed like, within three seconds, the nurse called me back. My mother stayed with me until they took me back for surgery. I only remember the nurse talking to me, telling me what to expect, and my doctor came in. He held my hand and told me that everything would be fine. He was going to take extra good care of me, and he promised I would not see any scars on my stomach.

He remembered our talk. I explained to him that I didn't want any scars on my stomach and didn't want to look like I had been butchered up surgically. I know that sounds very conceited.

However, I watched how they cut my mother during surgery and the awful scars it left on her body. I never wanted to experience that if I did not have to.

The doctor informed me that he would see me soon and the nurse would come back to put me to sleep. I remember the shot, my mother waving goodbye, kissing me on my cheek, saying I love you, and walking away. I remember rolling into the surgery room, my doctor smiling at me, and the lights went out.

The next thing I remember was waking up and looking at my mother holding my hand. The doctor came to let me know that everything went great. He would be back to talk to me more in detail tomorrow. I had to rest, and he had ordered medicine to help ease the pain. I informed him that I didn't have any pain.

He said, "That's great, but you will. Once the anesthesia starts to wear off, you will feel the surgery and be in some discomfort. Please push the white button when you start to feel the pain."

I remember going in and out. Awake one minute and asleep the next.

OMG...this sharp pain has awakened me out of my sleep. I thought that I was going to die from the pain. I pushed the white button and didn't let it go. I started to cry. The pain was too much to bear. It hurt to cry. It hurt to move. It even hurt to breathe. I have never felt pain like that before. The pain medicine finally started to work, and back to sleep I went.

The next thing I knew, the nurse was waking me up and letting me know I was being moved to my private room. My mother was in the room waiting for me. By this time, I am very hungry. I was told that I could only have liquid for the day and night. I could also try Jell-O if I wanted to. I really never liked Jell-O. However, I was so hungry that I was willing to try anything. I was able to drink some juice and a small amount of Jell-O. The pain started to die down some. However, I could feel the soreness of the incision.

It was now time for all visitors to leave the hospital, and my mother would have to leave. She will be driving my car and staying at my place. She informed me that she would be back bright and early in the morning to be here when the doctor came by. I said okay. She kissed me goodnight and left. I was feeling sleepy again and fell back off into a deep sleep.

I really could not get much sleep due to the nurses going in and out of my room all night checking on me. The next thing I knew, it was morning, and my mother was back in my room. Around 8:15 am, my doctor came into my room to talk with me. He informed me of how the procedure went, my healing timeframe, my therapy start date, and when I would be released from the hospital. I was informed that I would be in the hospital for one week, and I will start walking exercises today. I looked at my doctor in total shock and said, "What...are you serious? I have to get up out of this bed and walk today? Oh no, I can't do that." He informed me that I must, which would help me heal faster. He took a quick look around the surgical area, told me it looked good, and he will see me tomorrow.

After he left, within about ten minutes…the nurse came into the room to get me up to walk. I informed her that I would not be doing that. I feel it's too soon for me to be up walking. She informed me that I had to, or she will be forced to call my doctor. I told her to call him, and I didn't care. My mother asked her to please give us a few minutes and would she please come back in a little while. The nurse informed my mother that she would come back in thirty minutes. I informed my mom that I knew what she was about to say, and the answer was no. My mother began to reason with me and informed me that she knew for sure that walking was the best thing for me for a speedy recovery. I did not really feel what she had to say; however, I listened.

The thirty minutes was up now, and the nurse was back in my room. She informed me that it was time for me to get up and walk. During the process of me even sitting up in the bed, I thought I would die from the pain. When she tried to help me stand up, I screamed so loud that another nurse entered the room. I decided that it would be better for me to move around and get myself in position first to stand up, and then I would lean on her for support. After several minutes of taking my time to move about, I finally got my body positioned on the edge of the bed to stand up. I started to stand up, and it felt like everything from my surgery was coming apart. I leaned into the nurse crying a river and took one step. I had to stand there in that one step before trying to take another. My mother got on the other side of me, and I took the second step. Pretty soon, I was finally out of the room and into the hallway. I had to walk halfway down the hallway and back. It was a very slow and painful process.

I finally made it back to the room and into the bed. I was not in bed long before the nurse returned and told me it was time for me to shower. I had to get back out of bed and walk to the bathroom to do that. Here we go again. Pain seems to be my middle name right now. That was the slowest shower in my history books of showers. After my shower, I walked back into the room and got back into the bed slowly. Now, I am in a lot of pain. Pain medicine again and back to sleep.

I continued my daily walking exercises, and they became longer each day. By day three, the pain was not bad at all. On day seven, I was finally dismissed from the hospital with a six-weeks-at-home recovery period. My mother picked me up from the hospital, and we went home. She agreed to stay with me for the first four weeks of my recovery time. This would be hard for me. I had never been sick or down for a long period of time. I asked my mom to stop and get me some catfish and fries on the way home. For some reason, I just wanted to taste the food I couldn't eat while in the hospital. We stopped, picked up two meals to go, and headed home.

After arriving home, we ate and talked about my next steps. The food tasted so good while I was eating it. However, after I finished it, my stomach didn't agree with its contents. I paid dearly for eating that greasy fried food. Now I had two problems…my surgery pain and stomach pain. Why did I eat that food?

I decided to lie down in bed and try to go to sleep. I was sent home with medicine for pain. However, I have never been a fan of medicine and surely not a fan of prescribed pain medicine. I decided not to take anything for pain and tried to handle it with over-the-counter medicine. I finally fell asleep and didn't wake up until the next day.

Days and weeks start to go by very fast. It's time for my second doctor's check-up. During this visit, my doctor removes my stitches. He also removed the bandages; I would have to take care of the area myself and not get it infected. It has been four weeks, and my mother will leave to return to her home. Before she left, she ensured that I had enough food for the next two weeks. I will now be all alone. I was feeling good. I was convinced that I would be okay here by myself. I know my mother will only be a phone call away if I need her.

The remaining two weeks just flew by, and it's now time for my last doctor's appointment before I can fully be released from his care. My mother came over to drive me to my appointment. My doctor had not released me to drive on my own. I was so pleased with the incision. I could hardly see it, and it healed perfectly. My doctor informed me that everything looked good, and I was officially released from his care and free to drive myself.

Oh, happy day! I can finally start back living a normal life! I took my mother out to lunch as a thank you after my doctor's appointment and to celebrate! After our lunch, we did what I love to do…go shopping!!

> *"Heal me, O LORD, and I shall be healed; save me, and I shall be saved: for thou art my praise."*
> *~~Jeremiah 17:14 (KJV)*

Chapter 9

Married and Still No Child

*"The only impossible journey is the
one you never begin."*
~~Tony Robbins

I have been cleared by my doctor to drive and move about. However, I still feel a little sore from time to time. I am trying to take it somewhat slow. I would love to go out dancing. I better not think about doing that right now. I am really starting to be bored out of my mind. I am hanging out with friends somewhat. Not really a whole lot. Maybe the movies, lunch, dinner, and a little shopping.

It's only been about two weeks since I received a phone call from a friend. She and her husband are inviting me to dinner at their home. She also informed me that she had someone that they wanted me to meet.

I said, "Girl, really? I am still recovering from surgery. The last thing that I want to do is be introduced to some man right now. Besides, I don't like blind dates, nor have I ever been on one."

She continued to be very persistent in her request. She wouldn't take no for an answer. After weighing me down, I finally agreed to a dinner that would be in five days.

After accepting her invitation, I remembered how far she lived from me. This was going to be a very long drive for the first time after my surgery. I was not very excited at all. I didn't like blind dates and didn't want to be fixed up with anyone. For the remainder of the week, I kept trying to think of ways to cancel. I didn't want to go at all.

The day before the dinner, my friend informed me that we would be the only two single people at the dinner. *Everyone else is married. OMG...are you kidding me? This is getting worse by the day. I was literally in shock*!

Saturday is here, and it's time for the long drive to an unwanted blind dinner date. I arrive at my friend's home. All of the men are watching a football game. I didn't know which one he was.

My friend takes me off into one of her rooms to fill me in on all of the details. I reminded her that I was really not feeling this situation.

She said, "Relax. It will be fine, and you will like him." He is a really nice guy. In my world, a really nice guy meant boring.

Her husband called him into the kitchen and introduced us to each other. We both said hello, and he was smiling from ear to ear. I really was not attracted to him at all.

I learned that he really talked a lot. I actually thought that he talked too much. He began to ask me questions, and I gave him one-word answers. I was hoping it would turn him off, and he would leave me alone and stop talking to me. Instead, I think it turned him on. He would not stop talking and trying to get to know me better, no matter how bad I treated him. I started to think, *who is this guy, and why is he so into being treated badly by a woman he just met?*

It was time to eat dinner, and I tried my best to get away from him. However, I was not successful. He was always right by my side for the most part. He was very friendly and talkative. We all started to talk, joke, and have a great time. The time was moving fast, and I decided it was time to head home. I said goodnight to everyone and proceeded to leave. He followed me to my car and asked me if he could have my telephone number. I gave him my number, said goodbye, and drove home.

After arriving home, in less than thirty minutes, he called. He wanted to check to see if I arrived home safely. We talked for a while, and he asked if he could see me again. I thought I knew how I could get rid of him. I will tell him that he can come and go to church with me tomorrow morning. This was a Saturday night. He immediately said, yes and asked me what time would I like him to pick me up. Well, I was not expecting that response. I gave him the time and the address of my church. I didn't know him that well, and he was not coming to my home so soon. He lived over an hour away from me. However, he was willing to make the drive.

The next morning, he arrived early at my church. I was in total shock. We attended church together, and after church, we went out for lunch. We talked for a long time and got to know each other better. He was starting to seem like an okay guy. After lunch, we said our goodbyes and we both drove back to our homes. After he arrived back home, he called, and we talked some more. Well, one thing led to another, and we started dating. This was the third week of November. He decided to ask me to go home with him for Thanksgiving to meet his parents and family. Great, now that meant he had to meet my family. I told my mother about him. I wanted her to meet him and tell me what she thought. My mother had very good discernment of people. She agreed, and I brought him over to meet her that weekend. After watching her talk to him for a short time, I could tell she liked him immediately. That's a good sign coming from my mother.

My mother and family are very close. Now, I have to inform her that he asked me to spend Thanksgiving with him and his family in another state. We always spend holidays together, and I don't know how she will take this news. I decided to tell her over the phone later and not in person.

After leaving my mom's home, we returned to my place. He asked me when I was coming to visit him at his home. I informed him that he lived entirely too far from me. I really didn't want to drive that far to see anyone. However, I will make an exception since he is always driving to visit me. I decided to drive up to visit him at his home the following Saturday.

I got lost for a minute, but I finally made it there. He lived in a very nice home in a very nice neighborhood. I was impressed! I did inform him that I probably wouldn't be making this trip very often. This relationship is starting to progress very fast.

Well, it's time to tell my mother about my Thanksgiving plans. She was not happy at all. She asked if I had informed him that I was still recovering from recent surgery. I told her I had.

My mother said, "If a man still wants to be with you after he finds out that you just had surgery, he is a good person."

She still wanted to speak with him to let him know, I would be going with him this time. However, he better not ask me to leave my family again during the holidays. She then proceeded to give me her blessing and encouraged me to go.

Thanksgiving is upon us, and it's time for this five-and-a-half-hour road trip to meet his parents and family. He made sure that I had enough blankets and pillows. He suggested that I ride in the back seat to lie down. I'm really not a road trip person, and surely not more than five hours. This is the maximum that I will travel in a car.

The trip didn't turn out to be so bad after all. We arrived at his parents' home and had a great visit. I also met the rest of his family and ate lots of food! The time went by so fast. It's now time to head back home. It seemed like we arrived back home sooner than the trip down to his hometown.

The next day, I could feel the entire ride and trip in my body. I was very sore and really didn't do much that next day. We talked on the phone. However, I really didn't want any company. I just wanted to rest.

We continued to date and enjoy each other's company. The days and months are just flying by. It's now February, and he is asking me to marry him. Yes, I know that we just met each other in November. Well, I said yes, and we started to plan our wedding. But first, we had to pick out the ring. He wanted me to pick out the ring of my choice. It was the most beautiful and unique wedding ring I had ever seen. I loved it so much! Now the wedding planning can begin. We set a date for June. I know this all happened so fast. We said to each other…neither one of us is getting any younger! Only four months to plan a wedding. I knew that it could and would be done.

The planning went smoothly. It's now time for the wedding. It was small with family and close friends. We actually joked and laughed through the entire wedding ceremony. We were acting so silly and loving it! After the ceremony, we had a small reception. It was wonderful!

Now we are married, and it's time for me to move. We decided I would move to the city he was living in. The move went smoothly, and we now live together as husband and wife. We started trying to have a child right away. Nothing is happening. I am married and still have no child. Not even after my wonderful so-called fix-all surgery. *Did I go through that surgery for nothing? Will I ever really be able to have a child?*

"Wait on the LORD; Be of good courage, And He shall strengthen your heart; Wait, I say on the LORD!"~~Psalms 27:14 (NKJV)

Chapter 10

Excited - #Two

"Success is not final; failure is not fatal: It is the courage to continue that counts."
~~Winston S. Churchill

I was starting to get so discouraged, and then it happened. I took a pregnancy test, and it was positive. OMG…we were beyond excited. I decided that it was time to make a doctor's appointment to make sure. I was able to get in to see a new doctor in the area in which we were living from a referral within the week.

I took another over-the-counter pregnancy test, which was still positive. I can't stop praising God and crying at the same time. This was the happiest day of my life. I have waited for this day for so long. I won't be able to sleep until my doctor's appointment to truly confirm it's for real.

Well, it's time for my doctor's appointment. My husband was with me and drove me to the appointment. We arrived at the doctor's office and checked in. My name was called very quickly. I get into the room, and the doctor comes in immediately. He says to us. I hear we are pregnant. Let's check this out to be 100% sure.

He did an examination, took blood, and ran a urine test. It's official...we are pregnant! I started to cry again. I was six weeks pregnant. I was congratulated and made a second follow-up appointment in two weeks. I really didn't care for this doctor's personality. He didn't seem very caring at all. I was new to the area and desperate for a doctor. After the appointment, the drive back home was awesome. Talking about the pregnancy and thinking about the months ahead of us. Thinking about who we would tell first.

We arrived home, and of course, I had to call my mother first. She was so happy for me and said it was about time. We then called my mother-in-law and then my siblings. Next, I called my close friends. It was a great day!! I decided to cook because I just had so much energy. I couldn't wait until the next day to go to work and tell everyone.

During our morning meeting, I arrived to work and told everyone the great news. Everyone was screaming, jumping up and down, and congratulating me. I was so happy. Life was good, and I could not be happier. The weekend was here, and now it was time for church. I couldn't wait to get to church to tell everyone. Of course, we received the same reaction from our church family.

I started to make sure that I ate correctly and did all of the right things. I wanted to ensure that nothing went wrong and that I was doing my part to the fullest. I was always planning in my mind for the baby. I started to think about names and whether I wanted a boy or a girl.

One week, then two weeks, and now it's time for my second doctor's appointment. I am now eight weeks pregnant. My appointment went well. He also took a sonogram of the baby. Looking at that little dot in my stomach filled my heart with joy.

My doctor wanted me to come in every two weeks until I was twelve weeks pregnant. Off we go again, only to return in two weeks. I called my mother and filled her in on my doctor's appointment. She reassured me that I would be fine. Hearing her say that made me feel so much better. We laughed and talked until dark. After hanging up with my mom, it was late and actually time for bed. My husband and I have to be at work early in the morning. Life is still good, and I am the happiest that I have been in a long time. I wanted to pinch myself to see if it was really real. Sometimes, I actually thought that it was a dream.

My mind is racing 100 miles per minute. What should I do first? Should I start purchasing maternity clothes? Should I start shopping for baby furniture? Should I start setting up a room for the baby? What would we name the baby if it was a boy or girl? I knew inside that I was moving too fast with my thoughts. However, I was just so excited. I wanted everything to be perfect. I didn't want to forget any details. I started to ask God to please slow down my thoughts. I knew it was causing me to become stressed out, which was not good for me or the baby.

My prayer worked! My thoughts started to slow down and give my mind a little break. I continued going on with my life as normal. It's that time again, time for doctor's appointment number three. I am now ten weeks pregnant. My husband and I are on our way to the doctor's office again. We arrive full of joy and extra excitement. We will be able to see our little bundle of joy again today, I hope. My doctor started by listening to the baby's heartbeat. He started moving around my stomach with the stethoscope. He continued to go back and forth. I am starting to get worried. I asked the doctor if everything was okay. He said he was not sure, and he couldn't hear the baby's heartbeat. He wanted to do a sonogram as well. The nurse came in to set up everything for the sonogram. My doctor begins to do the sonogram. The same thing starts to happen again. He is moving the instrument back and forth on my stomach with a puzzled look. He then looked at me and said he could not find a heartbeat, and my baby was dead.

I could not believe what I had just heard. So uncaring with no compassion. My baby was dead. How could this be? What happened? Did I do something wrong? Are you sure? I had dozens of questions. I was in disbelief. This could not be true. Reality jumped in, and I started to cry uncontrollably. This was the worst day of my life. How could I be a mother one minute and then have my unborn child gone the next minute? No warning, nothing. The heart just stopped beating.

I asked to be along for a few minutes. This was too much to handle. The news weighed me down. I started to feel like I couldn't breathe. I couldn't speak. I just wanted to cry and call my doctor a liar. I didn't want to believe the news. I just cried and cried while my husband held my hands. He told me to stop crying and that everything would be alright. At that moment, I didn't feel anything would ever be alright again.

The doctor came back into the room and informed me that I must schedule a D&C to remove my unborn child from my womb. The nurse came in to schedule the procedure. It was scheduled for three days later at the hospital. I got dressed, checked out of my doctor's office, and left. This was truly the worst hurt that I had ever experienced.

The drive back home was silent. I didn't want to talk. I just wanted to get home and go to sleep. I felt that if I went to sleep, I would wake up, and this would all be a bad dream. Surely this cannot be happening to me. I am dreaming this for sure. I got right into bed with my clothes on. Something that I never do. However, I was in so much emotional pain that I didn't care about my clothes or anything else at that moment.

I slept for hours and didn't have an appetite. I finally woke up around 4:00 am. I got up and texted my supervisor at work to inform her that I would not be at work today. I went back to sleep until my husband woke me up around 7:00 am. He asked me if I needed him to stay home from work with me today. I told him no, I really wanted to be alone. I really didn't realize that he was in pain as well. I was so wrapped up in how I was feeling at the time. He went to work, and I stayed in bed all day and spoke to no one. I remember my supervisor calling me to find out how

I was doing and why I called in from work. I didn't answer the phone. I still didn't want to talk to anyone. My husband would call and check on me throughout the day. I would just answer the phone to say that I was okay.

I finally got out of bed to eat a little snack and got right back into bed. The pain hurt me so deeply. I just didn't feel that I could ever get over this. It was now 6:00 pm, and my husband was back home from work. He came straight into our room to check on me. I played like I was asleep because I still didn't want to talk about it. He let me sleep and continued to check on me from time to time.

On day two, he woke me up again at 7:00 am before he left for work. I texted my supervisor again and informed her that I would not be at work again and would call her once she arrived at the office. I realized that today I had to get up and face reality. I had to let my mother and my supervisor know what was really going on with me. I had to tell them today because the procedure was scheduled for tomorrow.

I waited and called my supervisor around 10:00 am, and she answered the phone. I informed her about my miscarriage and the procedure tomorrow, along with needing additional time off for healing after the procedure. She was very understanding and told me to take as much time as I needed. It was time to make the call I didn't want to make to my mother. I didn't want to tell her this very bad news. I didn't even believe that it was real. I called my mother and informed her of the news. She was very concerned and saddened that I didn't inform her for two days.

I told her I didn't want to and couldn't talk about it until now. I also informed her about the procedure in the morning. She wanted to be there with me. I told her that she didn't need to be there. My husband and I had to do this alone. She informed me that she did not like that she could not be there in support of me, but she would respect my wishes.

She told me that she loved me, and we said goodnight. I felt so alone and helpless. I felt like no one really understood the pain that I was feeling. It felt like my heart had been ripped out of my chest. I felt like I would never be happy again.

That dreadful day has finally arrived. It's time to go to the hospital. My procedure was scheduled for 8:30 am, and we had to arrive at the hospital at 6:30 am. Here goes another ride in silence. I felt so numb. It was so hard for me to actually believe that this was really happening. I fell asleep during the ride. Again, I hoped to wake up, and this would all have been a bad dream. I started to cry again. For some reason, as long as my baby was still inside me, I believed everything would be alright and things would change. I was dreading the procedure. That would finalize it all, and my baby would be gone forever.

We arrived at the hospital. I didn't want to get out of the car, but I had to. We walked into the hospital and checked in. I was called back shortly by the nurse and directed to a room.

The doctor came into the room shortly after we arrived. He wanted to check in to see if I had any additional questions before the procedure. He also informed me about the timeframe of the procedure, what would be done and what my recuperation timeframe would be. He seemed a little short, like he was in a hurry. I am not very fond of him. However, I didn't have another choice at this point. He informed me that I was about to be put to sleep and that I should say goodbye to my husband. I said goodbye, he kissed me, and out I went.

I remember waking up, feeling sleepy, and looking over to see my husband. The anesthesia started to wear off. I was wondering when the doctor was coming in to see me. He never came. The nurse informed me that I was being moved into a room. I started to feel sleepy again and fell back asleep. I was awakened by the nurse taking me to my room. While I was being rolled to my room, it felt like the medicine was wearing off, and I could start to feel some pain. After arriving in the room, I informed the nurse that I didn't feel very well. She started preparing me for the bed transfer and told me she would soon give me something for the pain.

Soon could not come fast enough. I was feeling my procedure now. It was starting to feel very painful. I pushed the button and also asked my husband to go and get the nurse. He came back with her. She informed me that she had been waiting for my doctor to contact her back. I was furious with my doctor. She finally installed the pain medicine and informed me when to push the button for release. It started to work immediately, and off to sleep again I went.

My husband woke me up in a few hours. He informed me that he was going home and would return early in the morning.

Off to sleep again I went. I was awakened often by the nurses to check my vitals. I was so out of it that I really didn't know what time it was. The next thing I knew, my husband was back at the hospital. It was 7:00 am. The doctor finally arrived at 8:30 am. I asked him why I didn't see him after my surgery. He informed me that he had another surgery after mine. I felt that was such an uncaring response to a patient. He told me that the procedure went fine, and he was sending me home. I really didn't feel like I should be going home. However, I didn't like him and would rather be at home.

The nurse came into the room while the doctor was still there. He gave her the instructions for my discharge. He left the room, and the nurse proceeded to help me get cleaned up and dressed. She then finished up my paperwork and gave me my instructions and prescription. My husband left to bring the car closer to the hospital and waited for the nurse to roll me out to the car. My husband and the nurse both helped me into the car.

She said, "Take care of yourself," and waved goodbye.

On the way home, my husband stopped at the pharmacy to fill my prescriptions. While waiting in the car, the pain started to flare up again. By the time we arrived home, I was in so much pain. My insides felt like someone had scraped them with a knife.

I started to bleed. I was in severe pain and scared to death. What was happening in my body? The doctor didn't tell me that I would feel like this. What did he do to me? I asked my husband to call the doctor. Something did not feel right.

He called the doctor's office, and they informed my husband that the doctor would call him back. He waited for one hour, and no callback. I called the doctor myself and asked to speak with him right away. I was not accepting him calling me back. I waited on the line for him for twenty minutes, and he finally got on the phone. I told him how I was feeling and everything that was going on with my body. He informed me that I was fine and not to worry. I was supposed to feel like this and bleed some. All of this was perfectly normal. I informed him that I was not bleeding some. I was bleeding a lot. He told me not to worry and hung up the phone.

I decided he would never touch me again when I recovered from this. I would not refer anyone to him. He was truly the worse doctor that I ever had. The way my body felt was proof enough for me that he handled it very roughly during the procedure. For several days, I was in so much pain and bleeding daily. I felt he didn't care, so I didn't call his office again.

The doctor's office called me to set an appointment for my follow-up after the surgery. I didn't want to see him again, but I had to. The appointment was scheduled for the following week. I continued to push myself to become strong and back to myself. I didn't take much of the pain medicine. I really don't like taking a lot of medicine. Every day I fought through the pain until I started to feel less and less pain.

Next week is here, and it's time for my check-up. I arrived at the doctor's office with my husband. When the doctor started my pelvic exam, I thought I would die from the pain. What did this man do to my insides? Why did it hurt so badly? I informed him over and over that it really hurt me. He seemed like he didn't care at all. He just kept telling me to relax. I started to cry. The pain from his examination was unbearable. I could not wait until he finished. I hated him, and I never wanted to see him again. He informed me that everything looked good, and I could return to work the following week. I checked out of his office, never to return. During my ride back home, I told my husband I must find a new doctor. I repeated that he would never touch me again.

We decided to stop and get something to eat. This would also get me out of the house for a few hours. It was good to be out of the house and feel somewhat better. I didn't know until the food arrived at our table that I was very hungry. I ate like it was my last meal and enjoyed every bite. My husband kept me talking, trying to keep my mind off the miscarriage. Reality set in, and my mind was thinking sad thoughts again. We finished our meals and headed back home. I became sad again and just wanted to go to sleep.

It's now a new day, and I must get back to normal. I started to prepare my heart and mind to return to work. That was something that I truly dreaded. I didn't want my co-workers asking me about the miscarriage and how I felt. I just wanted to be left alone. However, I knew that would not be the case when I returned.

Everyone was so understanding and caring. They really made me feel much better than I did before I entered the building.

Several of them wanted to take me to lunch, and I agreed. We had a great long lunch. I could surely get used to the long lunch part! Back to work we go. The day went by so fast. It's time to go home and do this all over again tomorrow.

"For his anger endureth but a moment; in his favour is life: Weeping may endure for a night, but joy cometh in the morning." ~~Psalm 30:5 (KJV)

Chapter 11

Nervous - #Three

"When you reach the end of your rope,
tie a knot in it and hang on."
~~Franklin D. Roosevelt

It's time to talk about finding a new doctor. I am unhappy with this new doctor and never want to see him again. I don't want to think about trying to get pregnant again until we find a better doctor. At this point, I don't know where to even start looking. I started asking ladies at work for recommendations. None of them lived close to me, which made their suggestions far from where I lived.

It's Saturday and time for me to go grocery shopping, as I do every two weeks on Saturdays! Upon arriving and walking toward the store, I ran into a lady named Angela. We both went to the same hairstylist. We hugged and started a conversation. I told her my situation and that I needed a good OBGYN. She informed me to look no further. She recommended her doctor for many years. She explained that he specialized in infertility, and she loved him so much. She informed me of her struggle with infertility and how her doctor helped her have several children. I asked her to please give me his info. She told me to call to schedule an appointment immediately and tell him that she had referred me to him. We said our goodbyes and I promised her that I would call him. I also told her that after visiting him, I would let her know my thoughts about him.

I returned home and told my husband about the doctor referral from a friend. I told him I would call on Monday to schedule a consultation with him. I was somewhat excited. I really hoped that I would like this new doctor. The previous doctor was awful. I pray that we never meet another doctor like him.

Monday has arrived, and I was on the phone with the doctor's office at 9:00 am sharp! I asked for a consultation appointment with him per my referral contact. I was able to get in to see him within the next two weeks. I thought that was too far away. However, I had to take what I could get. My appointment was scheduled for two weeks later at 8:30 am. I knew this would feel like the longest two weeks of my life. I informed my husband of the appointment date and time. That way, he could request time off to attend the appointment with me. I started praying that God would send us a good doctor. One that both of us would like. One who genuinely cared about women and childbirth. The next two weeks could not pass fast enough.

I called Angela to inform her of my appointment time as well. I told her that I would call her again after the appointment. The next two weeks moved so slowly. I thought the day of my appointment would never arrive.

Well, the day has come. It's the day of my appointment, and I am very excited. Praying that I would like this doctor, he will like us, and he will take me on as a new patient. We arrived at the office and checked in. I filled out the initial paperwork and waited to be called back to see the doctor. My name was called. My husband and I followed the nurse back into his office. We waited for the doctor to arrive. He entered the room, and my heart dropped. I became so nervous for some reason. He introduced himself to us and shook our hands. He began to make small talk with each of us. I began to hold a conversation with him. I really like his personality. It seemed like I had known him for years. We talked about Angela referring me and how long she had been a patient of his. We talked for about an hour. He informed me that if I wanted to have a child, he would do everything in his power, with God's help to make that happen. This was it, a doctor who loved the Lord. He asked me to have my medical records sent to him from my previous doctors and schedule a follow-up appointment after he receives the records.

We left his office with so much joy in our hearts. I really enjoyed my visit with him. He appeared to want to help me achieve my goal of becoming a mother. My husband really liked him as well. We both drove to work. Upon arriving to work, I immediately got on the phone with all of my doctors to request a rush order of my medical records. I told them I would come to their offices and pick them up. I scheduled them all and would have them all by the middle of the following week.

After receiving all the medical records, I drove them to my new doctor's office and scheduled a follow-up appointment. During this appointment, he would examine me and review my medical records with us. That appointment was scheduled for the following Monday morning at 11:00 am. I informed my husband, so he could be there with me. Upon returning to work, I informed my manager of my new doctor's appointment date and time. I also let her know what we are trying to do going forward.

The day of my doctor's appointment has arrived. We checked in and were called back immediately to see the doctor. He was waiting on us and greeted us while walking into his office. He started to go over each doctor's records and asked us questions. After the visit, he asked his nurse to come and take me to an examination room. I undressed and waited for the doctor to come in. My husband left and went back to the waiting area. The doctor and nurse entered the room. He examined me and took blood for lab work. I got dressed and went back into his office. He informed me that everything looked okay. However, I did have a lot of scar tissue from the tumor removal surgery. He stated that if we wanted to have a baby, we should go ahead and try again. I said, "Okay, we will," and exited the office. My husband and I went back to work. We would discuss our next steps and review what the doctor told us today later that night.

Over dinner, we talked about what we should do next. We both agreed that we should try again. Even though we were both scared and confused, we both wanted a child together. I must let go of my past fear and embrace the present. No one told me that I couldn't have a baby at this time. I've technically had my second miscarriage. I am able to get pregnant. Staying that way for nine months seems to be the problem.

We started trying to get pregnant again and live a normal life. Thinking about my past and not having that much hope. Well, it happened again very fast. I was pregnant again. We both were very happy. I made an appointment with my doctor to confirm that I was pregnant. My doctor's office got me right in to see the doctor. It was confirmed! I was six weeks pregnant, and everything looked fine. My doctor suggested that I come back for a follow-up in two weeks. I made the follow-up appointment and left. This was going to be the longest two weeks of my life.

We both went to work. I asked him to not tell anyone, including our family. I wanted to make sure before we told anyone this time. I broke the agreement on my way to work and called my mother. I had to tell someone. She was happy for me as always and assured me that everything would be okay this time.

I arrived to work and decided to tell my supervisor. I asked her to please not tell anyone. She promised. I had very bad concentration for the remainder of the day. I didn't really know how to feel. I was nervous about being excited. I didn't want to be let down again. I was half nervous and half happy.

After work, I stopped by the mall to look at baby clothes. That made me feel so much better. Oh, my, they have so many pretty things for babies, especially little girls! I can truly go broke in this store. I wanted my baby to have everything that I didn't have and more! I quickly snapped back into reality and realized it was too premature for baby shopping. I had to slow down and take it one step at a time.

I truly feel pregnant, which is a good feeling for me. I feel so positive now about this pregnancy. My body feels different this time. I told my husband that I felt much better about this one. We both started thinking, this just may be the one!

I am eight weeks pregnant now, and time to go back in for my check-up. My husband and I arrive at my appointment with smiles and anticipation! I'm called right back to see the doctor. We talk for a while, and then he does my sonogram. I didn't want to look out of fear. I just wanted to hear him tell me everything was looking great. He started to move back and forth, round and round on my stomach with the instrument. Lord, please, not again. He then asked me to look at the screen. Please, not this heart-dropping phrase again.

"Mrs. King, I am so sorry, but I don't hear a heartbeat from the baby."

My body goes numb again. I am in total shock again. Why is this happening again? My doctor stepped out of the room to give us a moment alone. My husband grabbed me in his arms as I cried. I cried so hard that I felt like I couldn't breathe. Why, Lord, why is this happening to me again? Why do my babies' hearts just stop beating? What's wrong with me? What's wrong with my body?

My doctor came back into the room to check on us. He gave us his condolences and informed me that I must have a D&C. I scheduled the D&C procedure for three days later and left to go home.

This has to be a dream. I cannot be going through this for the third time. Now, I have to give my mother the bad news again and my supervisor. I knew that I should not have broken our agreement. I told my husband that I told my mother and my supervisor. He informed me that he had also told his mother. We both had to deliver bad news.

After the D&C procedure, I went back into a period of depression. I could not understand why this kept happening, and no doctor could explain it. After long discussions and research, we decided it may be time to seek a second opinion from another specialist. I wanted my husband checked to ensure nothing was wrong with him and look into possible IVF treatment. The search begins for the right doctor. I received referrals from my present doctor. I assured him that it had nothing to do with him. I just wanted to check every area to see if I can find out why this keeps happening. He understood and wanted to help us in any way that he could.

"Wait on the LORD: be of good courage, and he shall strengthen thine heart: wait, I say, on the LORD." ~~Psalm 27:14 (KJV)

Chapter 12

Afraid - #Four

"Never let the fear of striking out keep you from playing the game."
~~Babe Ruth

We chose the first referral from our doctor and made an appointment. He was very booked up. However, my doctor called him to ask if he could squeeze us in sooner, and he did. We are scheduled to see him in one week. I decided to do research on him. I read nothing but good reviews and couldn't wait for our appointment. I decided to start writing down every question that I had for him. I didn't want to forget anything. I began researching possible reasons why this keeps happening to me to add to my list of questions.

The day of our appointment has arrived. I am so excited and afraid at the same time. So many questions are running through my mind. We arrived early. We are greeted with smiles and escorted right back to the doctor. He was actually in his office waiting for us. The initial contact was very pleasant. He seemed like a very nice doctor. He started with an interview list of questions for us. He had already reviewed my medical records and wanted to hear from us what we actually wanted to accomplish. I informed him that I wanted my husband and I to be tested. After the test results are back and depending on the outcome, I would also like to look into IVF and the cost. He informed us that he could start the process of testing us both during this appointment. I said, "That would be great. Let's get the ball rolling."

We completed the testing process. I was informed that he would have the test results in about two weeks. The testing consisted of checking my reproductive organs and my husband's. I felt like he was really attentive and made sure that he checked everything to get the answers that I so desperately needed. He also informed us that he would discuss the IVF process after receiving the test results.

We exited his office, not really knowing how to feel. That was a lot to take in for one day. Not knowing the outcome of the test was stressful. I was starting to think if all of this was really worth it. I was so tired after already having three miscarriages. Did I really want to possibly experience that again? What if I had another miscarriage? Would I be able to survive it? I was starting to become mentally drained. This was really taking a toll on my mental well-being. This has become all I think about… trying to have a baby. Meanwhile, my husband and I are still trying to work, act normal and work through a new marriage together.

The next two weeks could not come fast enough. Finally, it's time for our follow-up appointment to receive the test results. We arrive, and the nurse takes us right back to see the doctor. Again, he is waiting for us. We sat down, discussed current events, and got into the test results. He informs us that he can't see anything wrong with either of us. There is nothing that would prevent me from having a baby. I would just have to wait.

I was happy but still confused. I asked him if that was the case, why did I keep having miscarriages? He explained to me that the fact that I was getting pregnant meant that I could have a child. I would just have to wait for God's timing. Wow... he said, "God's timing." That meant that he was a man of God with much faith. I asked him about us doing IVR to help speed up the process. He informed me that he would not recommend it because he could not find any reason for the process. I said, "What if I wanted to do it anyway?" He said he could just take my money and perform the procedure to please me. However, he did not think it was needed and would not do it. I realized at that very moment that this doctor was on assignment to us by God. God was speaking through him very clearly...Not No, WAIT! We thanked him so much for everything. He asked us to schedule a follow-up appointment with my doctor, and he would also send the test results over to him.

We left the office in somewhat of a shock but also a sense of relief. Nothing was wrong with either of us. We just had to keep trying until God said yes! We both agreed from that very moment that we would not give up until God blessed us!

While driving back to work, I called my doctor's office to get the first appointment that I could. They were able to get us in within the next two days. We both are very blessed to have great jobs and very understanding managers. We arrived at our doctor's office to just go over the test results again and discuss our next move in this process. My doctor greeted us and asked how we felt about the appointment with the specialist. We informed him that we liked him and were confident in his results. My doctor stated that he agreed with the specialist after reviewing the test reports. Everything appeared to be in good order, and he couldn't see anything that would prevent me from having a child. We all agreed that we should keep trying if we were serious about having a baby. My husband and I agreed. We informed our doctor that even though I was somewhat afraid, we would try again. So, off we go, back to the trying to make a baby mood.

We both decided not to go back to work. We wanted to start trying again right away. We went home and well…you know the rest! We spent a great day and evening together. Not thinking about anything negative. It was only about us. We didn't think about anyone or anything during our day together! It was magical!!!

We went about our life as usual. Four weeks passed, and I realized I had not had a menstrual cycle. Off to purchase a pregnancy test. Took the test, and of course, it's positive. I tell my husband it's time to make a doctor's appointment. I can say that I'm not happy or excited this time. I am very afraid. We get to the doctor's office. The test confirmed that I was four and a half weeks pregnant. I really don't know how to feel. I should be happy. However, I have been let down so many times. I just could not be excited at all. I was afraid to be excited. We know the routine. We made an appointment for a follow-up in two weeks.

I told my mother again, and we waited. I informed my husband that I didn't feel very pregnant this time. It just didn't feel the same. I didn't know if it was because I was so afraid and didn't want to get my hopes up or if something was really different this time. I knew that I would find out soon enough.

The next two weeks seemed like one month. I never remember two weeks taking so long. I really wouldn't be surprised if my baby is gone again. For some reason, this pregnancy just doesn't feel like the others. I don't really feel anything at all. Maybe it was my way of protecting my heart from another disappointment. I really had a wall up this time. Mentally, I didn't feel or think that I was pregnant. I just wanted the time to go by, so I could get to the doctor and get this over with.

My husband and my mother asked me to stop thinking so negatively. I informed them that I had been through this three times already. I know my body, and I know when something just does not feel right.

It was time for my checkup. We arrive at the doctor's office and are called right back. My doctor talks to us for a while to see how we feel. I told him how I felt and wanted to get the examination over with. He said okay, and the nurse escorted us to an examination room. My doctor came in and started the examination. Before he could say anything, I told him, "No heartbeat, correct?" He looked at me and nodded. There was no heartbeat again. I didn't cry this time because I already knew it. I was not sad or angry like I normally was. My doctor asked me to get dressed and come back into his office.

After getting dressed, my husband and I went into my doctor's office. He told us how sorry he was that this was happening to us again. We talked about my next steps, which were, of course, another D&C. My doctor also informed us that due to the thinness of my uterus wall, I could have no more than five miscarriages'. After my fifth miscarriage, I would have to have a hysterectomy. That news took me by surprise. That meant if I got pregnant again and it was a miscarriage, that would be my fifth time. After that, if I had a sixth miscarriage, I would not be able to have another D&C. It would have to be a hysterectomy. That meant I would never be able to have children if I had to have a hysterectomy. That was truly a lot of information to take in. That sent me right back into depression.

I thanked my doctor for the information, scheduled the D&C, and walked out of my doctor's office in a daze. I could not believe the information that I had received. This had to be a nightmare. This cannot potentially be the end for me in trying to have a baby. I could not believe what I heard. My head started to hurt really bad. I just didn't want to do anything but lie down and be by myself. I was in total shock.

After arriving home, I went straight to my bedroom and got in bed with my clothes on. I was not hungry. I just wanted to go to sleep, hoping that this all would have been a bad dream when I woke up. I slept through the night and woke up around

6:00 am. I texted my supervisor, informed her that I would not be at work, and went back to sleep. I slept all day, only getting up to use the bathroom. I just didn't have an appetite or the energy to do anything. I was mentally drained. I was so tired of being disappointed and given bad news. For once, I was ready to receive something positive.

My mother was trying her best to help me feel better. I just couldn't snap out of that feeling of continuous disappointment. I was starting to think that being a mother was just not in the cards for me. Maybe, I have just been fooling myself into ever thinking that I would be a mother. Maybe God is punishing me for something I have done in my past? I was so hurt and confused.

It's time for another D&C procedure. I am so sick and tired of hospitals and D&Cs. The procedure went well, and back home I went to recuperate. While recuperating and letting my body heal. I needed to think hard about if I wanted to put my mind and body through this again. Am I doing the right thing by continuing to try and have a child? Am I just fooling myself about ever being a mother? I had to think long and hard about my future plans.

"I can do all things through Christ which strengthens me."
~~Philippians 4:13 (KJV)

Chapter 13

Broken - #Five

"The greatest glory in living lies not in never falling, but in rising every time we fall."
~~Nelson Mandela

While trying to act normal, I couldn't think about anything but if I should try again to get pregnant. If I do and I have another miscarriage, that will be it for me. I can't believe it has come down to this. I was so confused. I really don't know what to do. I started to think about adoption. I decided to discuss the process with my husband. He agreed if that was something that I wanted, he was in support of it.

We started to look for adoption agencies. After careful consideration, we decided on a particular agency. We had the initial interview, filled out the paperwork, and received the cost. We were in shock. We had no idea that it costs so much to adopt a child. However, we were willing to do whatever it took to have a child of our own. The search was on, and they would contact us after locating a newborn or infant child. We really didn't care about the sex of the child. We just wanted a healthy child to love and care for.

Two weeks have passed, and still no response from the agency. I was starting to get very stressed and worried. I wanted a child so badly. We decided to go to church on Sunday. The part of the sermon that caught our attention was about bringing a seed into your home that God did not send. That seed will bring you pain because you didn't wait and have faith in God. My husband and I freaked out. No one knew of our decision to try to adopt a child. We had not told anyone. Not even our parents or family. We knew immediately that was a sign from God to wait. We left church with a clear understanding that we should not follow through with the adoption process. We had to call the agency and withdraw our application.

The next day, we called the agency to inform them of our decision. Before I could inform her, she wanted to inform us that she had located an infant for us and wanted to send us a picture of her. OMG…we are now in shock. I asked her if we could call her right back. I hung up the phone in a daze. We had made a decision to resend our application. But now, she has located the one thing we have wanted…a newborn baby. We decided that we needed to pray about it. After we finished praying, there was such peace that fell upon both of us. We knew what we had to do. We had to continue with the withdrawal of our application for adoption. I called the agency and informed them of our decision. She begged us to reconsider. I informed her that we had decided to wait on our blessing from God.

She asked us to please think about it a little longer, and she would call us back in a few days. I told her that she was welcome to call us back; however, our mind was made up. The peace of God was all over me for the first time. I felt God would bless us if we kept that faith and did not give up on God. We decided that we should try again to have a child.

The journey begins again. We start trying to have a child. Weeks go by, and I start to feel sick to my stomach. I decided to take a pregnancy test, and again it was positive. Here we go again. I made the doctor's appointment for confirmation. After my appointment, it was confirmed. I am eight and a half weeks pregnant again. I have faith, and we truly believe God will bless us this time. I don't feel worried or afraid at all. My check-up was good. Now it's close to Thanksgiving. We drove up to LA to visit my in-laws for the Thanksgiving holiday. We were not going to tell anyone that I was pregnant. Of course, you know that I told my mother.

This was going to be a five-and-a-half-hour ride, both ways. We began to prepare for the trip, and I noticed that I would start to get tired more quickly. I thought to myself, this is how I was supposed to feel while being pregnant. I became happy and full of hope. On the road we went. I spent most of the trip in the back seat to rest. The trip went well, and I was feeling pregnant. We arrived safely and had a great time with family. It was time to head back home. We packed up the car, said our goodbyes, and off we went.

I decided to sit in the front seat for our drive back home. It started to rain very heavily. About two hours into our drive home, I started to feel cramping pain. I had never felt that before. It started to get worse and worse. It was very painful. Finally, I could not take it anymore. I asked my husband to stop at the next restroom that would be clean. We stopped at a Kroger grocery store. I told my husband I would be fine and went into the store alone. I went straight to the restroom. The pains became sharper. I knew something was wrong but didn't know what it was. All at once, it felt like I really needed to urinate. I started to use the restroom, and it didn't feel like urine. I turned around and looked into the toilet and saw my baby fetus in the toilet. I had another miscarriage. Only, this time, it came out on its own. I just stood there in the bathroom stall and cried. I hated to flush the toilet. I felt like I was just flushing my baby away. It took me a while to get my emotions intact.

My phone began to ring. It was my husband. I answered the phone and told him that I would be out shortly. I cleaned myself up and continued to stare into the toilet. I could not get that vision out of my head. I could actually see that it was a baby. I realized that day that I was stronger than I ever thought would be possible. I really thought that I was going to lose my mind that day. However, God gave me the strength to straighten myself up, flush the toilet and walk out of that store in one piece.

I got into the car, and my husband had many questions. I remember turning around, looking at him, and saying, "The baby is gone." I began to tell him what had happened. I could see the hurt, shock, and disbelief in his eyes. He asked me why I did not call him into the store. Why did I go through that alone?

I really couldn't answer his questions. I just knew that it was something that I had to do alone. Besides, he could not go into a ladies' restroom with me.

The drive home would become extremely long and painful. Very few words were spoken. I cried a lot during the entire ride home. I was so broken. It could not get any worse than this. This cut straight through my soul. I had no more fight in me. I felt so weak and helpless. I finally cried myself to sleep. My husband woke me once to see if I wanted anything to eat or needed to stretch my legs. I just wanted to sleep. We continued with the long journey back home.

We arrived home, and my husband woke me up. I just walked out of the car, straight to our bedroom, and got in bed. I didn't want to talk or eat. I just wanted to sleep this pain away. While lying in bed for a short while, I realized that I couldn't sleep. My mind started to race. What happened? Did I do something wrong? How could this happen? Why did it happen this way? My head started to hurt. I had so many unanswered questions. I decided to call my doctor and tell him what had happened. He informed me to call the office in the morning, and they would get me in to see him. He assured me again that I was going to be alright. I tried to go to sleep, but I just couldn't sleep. I decided to get out of bed, fix myself something to eat, and watch television. While watching television, I started to talk to God. I asked Him why. What did I do wrong? Why does this keep happening to me? I cried out to God. I told Him that I could not go through this again. I am so tired and broken. I just can't survive this type of hurt and pain again. This was all that I could take. I cried out to the lord and fell asleep praying.

I woke up the next morning on the sofa, still in my clothes. I called my supervisor to inform her that I was not coming to work. I then called my doctor's office to schedule an appointment. I was informed to get there ASAP, and they would fit me in. I informed my husband, took a shower, and changed my clothes. Off we went to the doctor's office. We arrived and were taken right back to my doctor's office. My doctor came in shortly and told us how sorry he was. He needed to examine me to ensure that I had a miscarriage. He wanted to be sure that the fetus was no longer inside my uterus. We proceeded with the examination. The results showed that I had a miscarriage, and the fetus was no longer in my uterus. The good news was that I would not have to endure another D&C procedure.

After getting dressed, my doctor wanted to talk to us again before we left his office. He encouraged us that before we give up, we should still try again. He knew that it would be difficult for me. However, he felt that God was going to bless us. We prayed in his office and left. This was something that I really didn't feel like even thinking about at that time. I knew that I didn't want to go through that again, ever in life.

> *"The Lord is close to the brokenhearted; he rescues those whose spirits are crushed."*
> *~~Psalms 34:18 (NLT)*

Chapter 14

I Need a Miracle

"All you need is one YES from God!"
~~Tyler Perry

It's time to tell my mother again for the 5th time that I had another miscarriage. I began to sound like a broken record. My mother, at this point, was very worried about me. She replied with a statement that I was not expecting. My mother told me I should stop trying to have a child before I killed myself. She also said that having a child is not all that it seems. I was so hurt by her reply. I responded, "That is easy for you to say, mom. You have five children. Right now, I am just trying to have one child."

I had to say goodbye to my mother and hang up the phone. I really could not believe that she had said that to me. I know she is afraid for me, but that statement coming from her cut me very deep. I begin to doubt what I should do. I talked to my husband about what my mother said to me. He assured me that my mother meant no harm. She just loves me and is very concerned about my health. He asked me if I really wanted to try again. I was not sure at that point. We decided that we should pray about it again. I decided to spend hours daily in prayer to God for direction. I needed to hear from him before I went any further. I spent lots of time in prayer to God. At this point in my life, I developed a strong prayer life. I cried out to God daily. It was all about me and God. Nothing else really mattered. I had to hear clearly from God.

After several months of prayer, I informed my husband that the Lord told me to try again. I had such a wave of peace upon me this time. I had never felt this kind of peace. I had peace that whichever way the next pregnancy turned out, I would be okay, and it would be God's will for my life. My husband informed me that he felt the same way and we should try again. Here I go again…trying for the sixth time!

As usual, it didn't take long before I became pregnant again. We decided this time to not tell a soul. We would only tell our managers at work. Only because we would both have to take off work for doctor appointments. We made the appointment to see my doctor for formal confirmation. It's official, we are pregnant again. I am excited, nervous, afraid, and broken…all at the same time. If it turns out to be another miscarriage with no heartbeat, I will have to have a hysterectomy. That meant no future chance of me carrying and having my own child.

I prayed like never before. I was reading the word of God daily. I could not get enough of reading God's promises to me. I started to pray God's word back to him. I was 39 years old and pregnant. I loved reading about how God blessed Sarah in Hebrews Chapter 11. I would find myself daily telling God… **"I know that you didn't love Sarah more than you love me. If you** *bless me with a child, I will be a good mother. I will raise this child up to know and love you. I will dedicate my child back to you."* This was my daily plead to God. I would ask Him daily to bless me like He blessed Sarah in her old age.

I'm feeling pregnant now. Having a mild case of morning sickness. Overall, I am feeling pretty good. It's time for my first check-up, and I am so nervous. This will be my 8-week check-up. The check-up went well. I am scheduled to return in two weeks. I will be okay if I can just make it to 12 weeks. I have never made it that far.

I am working and trying to act normal and not let on that I am pregnant. I noticed that I'm getting a little tired from time to time, and I am not really doing that much. My focus is a little off at work. My mind can't think of anything but making it to 12 weeks of pregnancy and the continued heartbeat from each check-up. The days at work seem so long. I didn't want to be there, but I had to work. If I was just sitting at home, I would probably go insane.

It's check-up time again. I am now at 10 weeks. My doctor decided to let me hear this time. This has been a bad visit in the past. We both braced ourselves for this check-up. Immediately, when my doctor started the sonogram…we could hear a very strong heartbeat. OH, LORD JESUS! This was the best sound that we had ever heard. I was so happy that I could not stop crying. We scheduled my next two weeks' appointment and left the office. My doctor said that he felt very good about this pregnancy. I replied, "Only time will tell."

I decided that now it was time to talk to my baby. I started reading the bible out loud to my baby. I played gospel music and placed the speakers on my stomach. I told my baby all day and every day how much I loved (him or her). I wanted them to hear the word of God and develop love from the womb for God and music.

I would tell my baby, "Mommy needs you to stay with me. I love you, and I need you in my life. Please fight for mommy. Please don't leave me. I love you so much. I can't wait to see you and show you just how much I love you."

I wanted my baby to feel the love that I had for them. I needed them to feel that love in the womb. I thought that if they could feel the love, it would give them a reason to fight and develop properly.

Well, it's time for my 12 weeks check-up. I was so nervous that I had a headache from fear. During the examination, I turned my head. I could not bear any more bad news. My doctor informed me that the heartbeat was still strong, and everything looked great! I am now 3 months pregnant. OMG… I have finally made it past the risky stage. I am on cloud nine. I am so happy and could not contain myself. We can now tell all of our family and friends.

My doctor informed me that because of my age...he would like to do a sonogram each month to monitor the baby and me carefully. We scheduled my next appointment and went to lunch to celebrate!! This was one of the happiest days of my life. I could not believe that I was three months pregnant. I felt extremely hungry and ate like a pig. The excitement brought on my appetite. My husband and I had a great lunch together and could not wait to get home and share our good news with everyone!

During our drive home, I called my mother to inform her of the exciting news! She was so happy for us. She reminded me to take good care of myself and the baby! When we arrived home, I had already contacted and shared the good news with my immediate family! This was a long-awaited moment for my family. After we arrived home, we contacted my supervisor and a few of our close friends. We couldn't wait for church service on Sunday.

I started a daily routine with my baby. I would talk to my baby all day. I told my baby how much I loved it. How much I needed it in my life. How they have been created with love. How I can't wait to see them and kiss all over that beautiful face. How they will be my gift from God! I would have devotion time with my baby daily that included music, scriptures, prayer, and conversation. I would go into the guest bathroom in my home daily and spend that time with my child and God. I still, to this day, do not understand why I chose the bathroom, but I did.

Life was good. People treat you so nice when you are pregnant. I was enjoying every second of my pregnancy. I started to have the weird food craving while driving my husband crazy with the store runs. I didn't gain a lot of weight during my pregnancy. I felt great! My doctors' appointments are going great. No problems at all. Reviewing my child's sonogram monthly and seeing the actual development was life-changing.

I am five months pregnant and at the point of finding out the sex of the baby. I wanted to know; I could not wait. It was really hard to find out the sex. This child was very stubborn and didn't want to be bothered during this time. I realized that daily around 12:30 pm was him/her nap time. They did not want to be bothered at all. I remember that little face looking at us with disgust and moving its body very quickly. That was to say…you better get this photo on the first try because I am not moving again. My doctor got the shot, and IT'S A GIRL!!! I am so happy. I really wanted a girl deep down inside. I am crying tears of joy! My doctor informed us that the birth would be on January 28, 2000. I had to have a cesarean section to play it safe. This is also the birth date of my father!

Another good day! I am so happy and still in awe of God's love for me. The enemy tried to make me feel like this day would never happen for me. But God said yes! Praising God all the way back to work. I called my mother and informed her before going into the office. After arriving in the office, I shared my sonogram with my co-workers. We all cried together and hugged each other tightly. They were so happy for us, and I thank God for each of them.

Baby showers are starting to be scheduled and planned. This is really happening. I am having a baby girl! God is so good! I have been informed about FIVE baby showers scheduled for me. I had never heard of anyone having that many baby showers. Two showers were given by my job/co-workers. One was given by my friends. One was given by my church, and one by my family and close friends. Oh my God…this baby is blessed and highly favored by the Lord. I couldn't wait to tell my husband about this good news. He was just as surprised about the five baby showers!

Things are going so well. I am the happiest that I have ever been in my life! We are shopping for baby things and started to purchase baby furniture and set up the baby's room. Shopping for a girl is so much fun. They had so many beautiful things to buy for baby girls. I was like a kid in a candy store. So much to choose from. This part of the process was more fun than I could have imagined! We had a great time purchasing and preparing for the arrival of our baby girl. We had already decided on her name. Alexis Renee King. She will have my middle name! Things are going good and according to plan. We are so happy!

Well, as the old saying goes…the enemy is always present, and I am about to find that out the hard way. We arrive back home. I am in the office, and my husband is in the family room. I pick up our home phone in the office to call my mother. When I picked up the phone, I heard a woman's voice on the other end of the phone, saying that she really enjoyed their time together in the park. She hated leaving, but she forgot her glasses and needed to go and get them. I was in total shock. Did I hear her correctly? Did a woman just say that she has been in a park today with my husband? When did this happen today? Is my husband cheating on me while I am pregnant? I continue to listen to him navigate through his voicemail messages from his cell phone. I decided to place the phone on the desk and walk into the family room. He immediately knew that I had heard his message.

"Are you having an affair on me while I am pregnant?"

"No."

I walked closer to him and asked him again. But this time, I knew that my facial expression was looking enraged.

"She was just a friend from work."

The questions from me kept coming, and he kept lying. I knew he was lying. At this point, one of the sayings that my mother would tell me came to mind. You never have to leave your home to find out if someone is being deceitful. Just keep an intimate relationship with God; He will bring the evidence to you and lay it in your lap.

I immediately had to snap out of this situation. The stress could hurt my baby and cause me to have a miscarriage. As I walked toward our bedroom, I could not believe what I had just experienced. This could not be real. This is not happening now. Why Lord? How could he do this while I'm pregnant? Lord, why did you let him do this to me? We both prayed for this child. He knows this type of stress could cause me to have a miscarriage.

I started to cry uncontrollably. I didn't think he would do such a thing. What did I do to him that would make him do this? What kind of woman would be with a married man with a pregnant wife? This was all too much for me to handle. I was pregnant and now thinking about divorce. I asked my husband to leave the house. However, he told me that he was not leaving.

As the days went by, I really started to hate my husband for what he did. I decided that I was going to divorce him. But before I made that final decision, my mother asked me to try and talk with him about it. So, I did just that. He became very disrespectful verbally during the conversation. He told me to my face that he liked the other woman and would like to be with both of us. At that very moment, I think that my whole body went into shock. He had the nerve to say that to me. I told him at that moment that I wanted a divorce. He stated that if that's what I wanted, he was okay with it. I told him that I would move forward.

The next day I told everything to my mother and informed her that it was over. This is something that I always said that I would never put up with. First of all, my husband knows I would have left him if he had tried this before I was pregnant. Secondly, the enemy knows how much I wanted a child, and now that God has blessed me, he was trying to make me lose my unborn child and cause my child to be born into a broken home.

My mother stated that my child had a calling on their life from God and that the enemy does not want that calling to come forth. My mother asked me to please think and pray about it before making any final decisions.

I tried to move forward with my life. It was so hard. My husband and I argued all the time. At this point, I didn't believe or trust him at all. I prayed and asked God for help and direction. I didn't want to move on my own understanding. I just needed guidance, direction, and peace.

The next day, a friend called me out of the blue. We had not talked to each other in a while. She called to say that God had placed my name on her heart. She had a book that she was supposed to give to me. The book was titled: The Power of a Praying Wife by Stormie Omartian. I said okay, and she asked if she could drop the book off at my home. I informed her that I would be at work during that time. She asked if she could place it on my front porch. I agreed.

I arrived home from work to find the book on my front porch. My first thought was, please, I do not feel like being a praying wife right now. Surely, the Lord does not expect me to pray for my husband. The only prayer I wanted to pray for him was please, Lord, don't let me hurt him, go to jail, and leave my child without a mother.

I started to read the book; it was a pretty good read. I was enjoying the book until I got to the part about praying for my husband. Hold up, wait a minute. Why should I pray for him? He is the one that should be praying. I didn't like or understand that part at all. God started to work on me. He reminded me that praying for my husband would heal me and set me free from my hurt and anger. It took me days to finally surrender and pray for him.

After praying for my husband, I noticed that I started to feel better. I received my self-worth back. I no longer felt like something was wrong with me. I realized that I needed to get my heart and mind right with Christ and for my unborn child. I finally understood the attack from the enemy on my unborn child. My attention began shifting from my husband to the one attacking my marriage and my family.... SATAN. I became very angry and ready to fight back.

It was time for me to tell him who the boss was. I had to let him know that he would not hurt my unborn child. He could not have my marriage or my husband. He was not going to stress me out, pour stress into my child's spirit, or cause me to have a miscarriage. I am taking back control of my life and my marriage.

I started to pray for my husband daily and asked God to forgive him and show mercy upon his life. My baby shower dates are approaching, and I am very excited. I am going to enjoy my blessing from God. I refuse to let any demon from hell destroy the blessings God has stored up just for me. I will enjoy every moment of this time of pregnancy and becoming a mother!

I attended all five baby showers, and my husband has attended with me for the most part. We are moving right along. I have spoken with him and laid down the ground rules for this family. He followed the rules, and I didn't have to repeat myself. After attending the last baby shower, we had enough diapers for our baby girl for one whole year. Her closet was full to the top of the ceiling with diapers. God is so good to us! I never dreamed that God would bless us like this. I knew that I would not be delivering an ordinary child. God had big plans for her life. That is why the enemy hated her so. She had favor with God and man!

My husband started to inform me that he noticed a big change in me. I informed him that I had been praying for him, our child, and our marriage. I have also turned him over to God and dedicated our daughter back to the Lord.

> *"For all of God's promises have been fulfilled in Christ with a resounding "Yes!" And through Christ, our "Amen" (which means "Yes") ascends to God for his glory."*
> *~~2 Corinthians 1:20 (NLT)*

Chapter 15

My Gift from God

*"Man gives you the award,
but God gives you the reward."*
~~Denzel Washington

I continued to praise, pray, and worship God for my miracle. I was determined to not let the enemy steal my joy any longer. My child will be born healthy and happy! I continued to work. However, I was just not feeling like going into the office anymore. I am now in my eighth month and starting to feel tired. I decided that it was time for me to go on leave from my job. I asked my doctor to send the request to my employer.

I am now at home enjoying my pregnancy and waiting for our child's delivery date of January 28, 2000! I can't wait to see her and tell her that daily. I continued to read God's word to her, play worship/gospel music against my stomach, and talk to her all day. Time is moving fast, and I am ready to see her and get my body back.

Well, it's time! The awaited day has arrived. I am so nervous. My mother and sister are with me. It's a snowy/icy day. I am so afraid that we could have an accident on the way to the hospital and my unborn child will be hurt. So many emotions are taking over me on this day. I am happy, nervous, and afraid all at the same time. My husband is taking his time and driving very safely. I started to pray and ask God to calm my spirit.

We arrive at the hospital safely and on time. I was taken back immediately and prepped for a C-section. During my vital check, I was told that my blood pressure was very high. I have never had any problems with my blood pressure before. I became stressed all over again. I was worried that my elevated blood pressure would hurt my baby and that I would not be able to deliver her today.

My doctor came into the room, calmed me down, and ensured me that I would have my healthy baby today and he would get my elevated blood pressure stable first. I felt so much better because I truly trusted my doctor. I knew he wanted only the best for us and would do everything within his power to deliver our child safely. The next thing I knew, my blood pressure was normal, and I was being taken back for delivery. My mother, sister, and husband kissed me goodbye.

I arrive in the delivery room, and the process begins. I am awake during the delivery. I could not see anything, but I could somewhat feel the process. My baby has arrived! I saw her being raised in the air and given to the nurses. That wonderful cry that you are waiting to hear happened. I wanted to see her so bad. All of a sudden, I could not breathe. I felt just like I was dying. My eyes started to roll back inside of my head, and I couldn't speak to tell the nurse behind me. Everyone was looking at the baby. Just when I felt I was leaving this world, the nurse put the oxygen mask back on my face. I was able to breathe again and felt so much better.

By this time, my baby had been cleaned up, and they gave her to my husband first. He just held her and looked at her with so much love in his eyes. He would not take his eyes off of her. I finally asked if I could hold my baby. The nurses took her from my husband and gave her to me. She was the best thing that I had ever laid eyes on. She was just perfect to me. I cried hard, kissed her multiple times, and told her how much I loved her and how happy I was to finally see her. It was truly love at first sight. Of course, I never loved anything or anyone as much as I loved her after God.

My baby was then taken to the nursery, and I was placed in a temporary room. My family was now able to come in and see me. They brought my daughter to me. My mother, sister, and I cried over my blessing from God. My daughter never went to sleep like most newborn babies. She was still awake, looking at us and holding up her head. My mother said, "This is going to be a smart and curious child."

I was soon moved into a private room. They brought my daughter back into the room with me. We informed the nurse of her name Alexis Renee King. I was in the hospital for one week and then released to go home. During my one-week stay, I had so many visitors and flowers in my hospital room. I felt so loved and blessed. I couldn't wait to leave the hospital with my bundle of joy and start being her mother!

It's time to leave the hospital. I rode home in the back seat with her. I could not take my eyes off her. She was the sweetest sight that my eyes had ever seen. Oh, how in love I am with her. I never knew that I could love any human being like I love her. Words cannot explain how you feel after bringing a life into the world. It is truly a gift that only God can give you! I am inside the house now and still holding her. I just can't lay her down. Oh, how long I have waited for this day. I just can't stop looking at her, crying and thanking God...all at the same time.

Life is good, and I love being a mommy! My husband and I discussed her future. I decided that I wanted to spend every moment enjoying being her mother. I wanted to be there for every FIRST that she had. I decided to quit my job and become a full-time mom! My mother was at my home helping me with Alexis for the first month of her life.

It was time for my mother to go back home. The next day she had her routine doctor appointment. During her appointment, she was informed that she needed to have surgery, which involved placing a stent in her heart valve. I was very against the procedure and not a fan of her doctor. I asked her to please get a second opinion. She loved her doctor and believed anything that he said. Against my wishes, my mother proceeded and scheduled the surgery.

I was so tired from being a new mom and dealing with my marital problems. I just didn't have any fight left in me at that moment. I was not happy at all, but I didn't have the energy to go back and forth with her on the issue. She informed me of the date and time of the surgery, and I assured her that I would be there.

I was there with her during the surgery while trying to take care of a newborn baby. I was told that the surgery was a success, and my mother would go home in one day. I thought that was very soon, but her quack doctor tried to ensure it would be okay. My mother was released from the hospital on Wednesday, following her surgery on the previous Monday.

I was there to drive my mother home from the hospital and made sure that she had everything that she needed. I stayed with her for two days and returned home early that Friday morning. My husband and I made plans to drive to visit his mother and take Alexis to see everyone on his side of the family.

I arrived home and began to prepare for our departure road trip to LA. Suddenly, while packing, I heard a voice say, "Stop packing and stay home." What? I don't understand. It spoke to me again, and I knew then that it was the Holy Spirit speaking to me. I didn't know why or understand, but I obeyed.

My husband was packing up the car. I had to call him into the house and tell him that I wouldn't be going out of town with him. He was furious! He said, "Okay, I will take Alexis with me so my family can see her."

Of course, the answer to that was no. My newborn baby wasn't going anywhere without me. This became a huge, escalated argument that turned into him calling his mother. She tried to talk me into coming as well. I told her I could not come and didn't know why. I was very sorry.

My husband went ahead and took the trip without us. After he left, I called my mother to inform her that we hadn't made the trip and would be over to visit with her in the morning. My mother asked me if we could come over now. My mother lived an hour from us, and it was already late. I informed her that we would get up and drive early in the morning. She continued to ask me to come now. However, I kept telling her that it was late and that we would see her in the morning. We talked for a little while and said goodnight.

The next morning, I woke up early and got things together for our drive and visit to my mom's. I called her around 8:00 am and received no answer. That was strange, but I knew she sometimes went walking early in the mornings. I waited and called her again around 9:00 am, and still no answer. This is not normal, and I am now feeling a little uneasy. I decided to call my brother, who now lived in the same city as my mom. I asked him if he had spoken to mom this morning. We all talked to her every day. He stated that he had called her earlier with no answer. We talked for a while and decided he better go over to her home.

My brother arrived and called to tell me he was there. However, he could not get into her home with his key due to the deadbolt lock. That only happens if she is in the house. We are now very concerned. He informed me that he would have to break the window to get in and call me back. I waited for a few minutes and called my brother back with no answer. I called him back several times, and still no answer. I am shaking at this point. This does not feel good at all. Minutes later, my brother called me back crying and telling me that our mother is gone. With unbelieve, my first response was gone where? He informed me that our mother was dead. He found our mom in the bathtub underwater. She was taking one of her hot baths, as she always loved to do while painting her fingernails and eating grapes.

I felt my heart stop beating for a second and was numb. Alexis started to cry, and that made me snap back into reality. Now, I understood why I could not go on that trip with my husband. The Lord knew I could not have taken this kind of news out of state. I needed to be at home with my family. This was one of the saddest days of my life. I had lost my mother and best friend. I also had a newborn baby and no one to help me with her. I called my husband to inform him of my mother's passing. He informed me that he was on his way back home.

I had to break down and call a friend to come over and take care of Alexis for me while I went to comfort my family and start making arrangements for our mother's funeral. I thank God that I was able to have pictures of my mom with Alexis. I lost my mom right before Alexis turned three months old.

Well, the rest is history! Alexis is now a college graduate as of May 7, 2022. This was also my late mother's birthday! I know my mother would be so proud of her and happy that she graduated from college on her birthday! I truly know firsthand about this scripture: *"The LORD gave, and the LORD hath taken away; blessed be the name of the LORD" Job 1:21b (KJV).*

*"**Now this is the confidence that we have in Him, that if we ask anything according to His will, He hears us.**"*
*~~1 John 5:14 (**NKJV**)*

Alexis from Conception through 22 years old

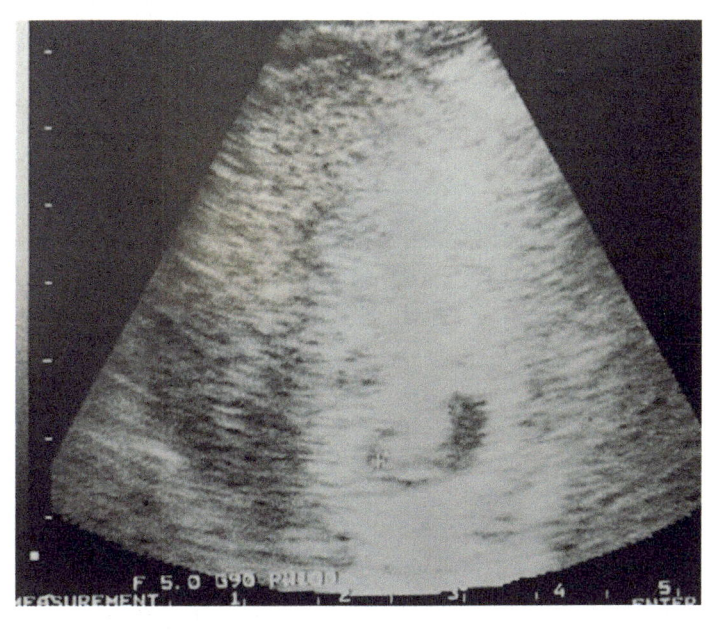

Alexis' sonogram at 7 weeks and 4 days

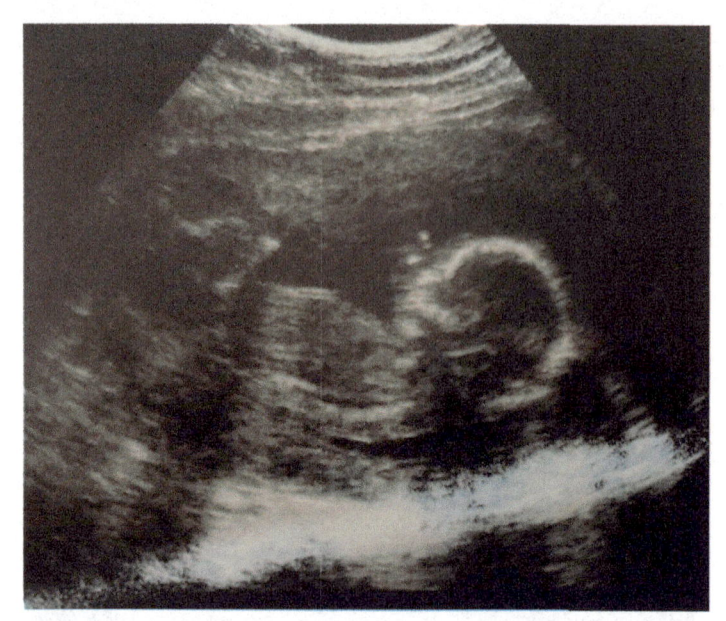

Alexis' sonogram at 4 months

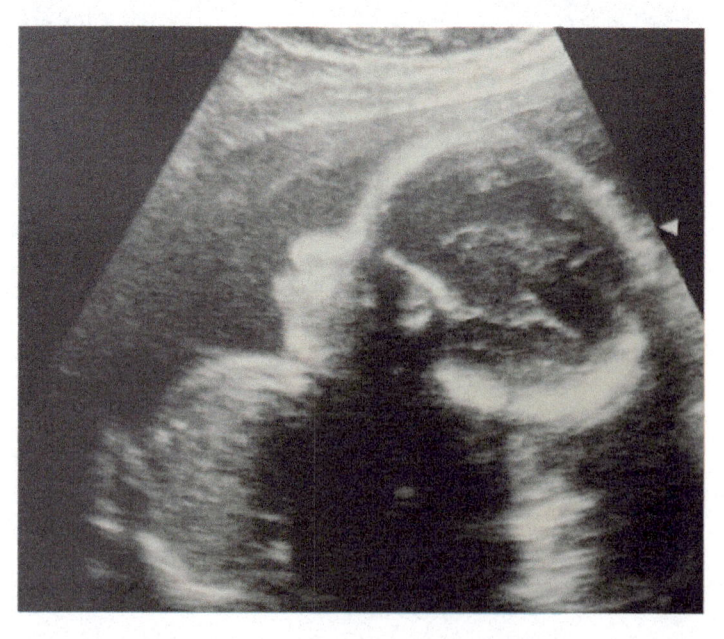

Alexis' sonogram at 7 months

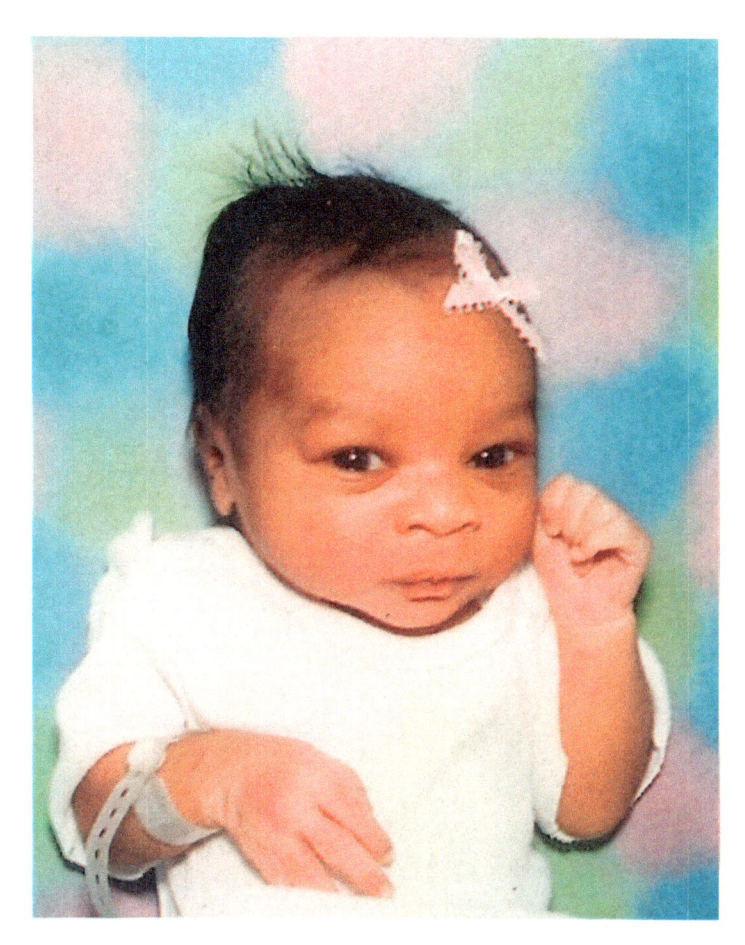

Alexis at Birth

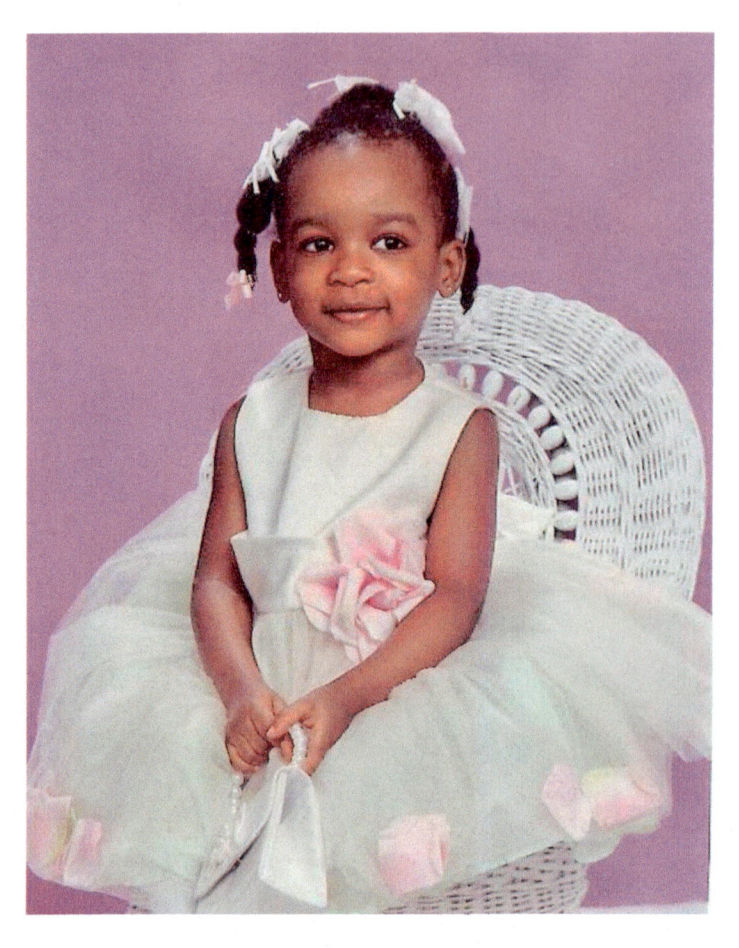

Alexis at 3 years old

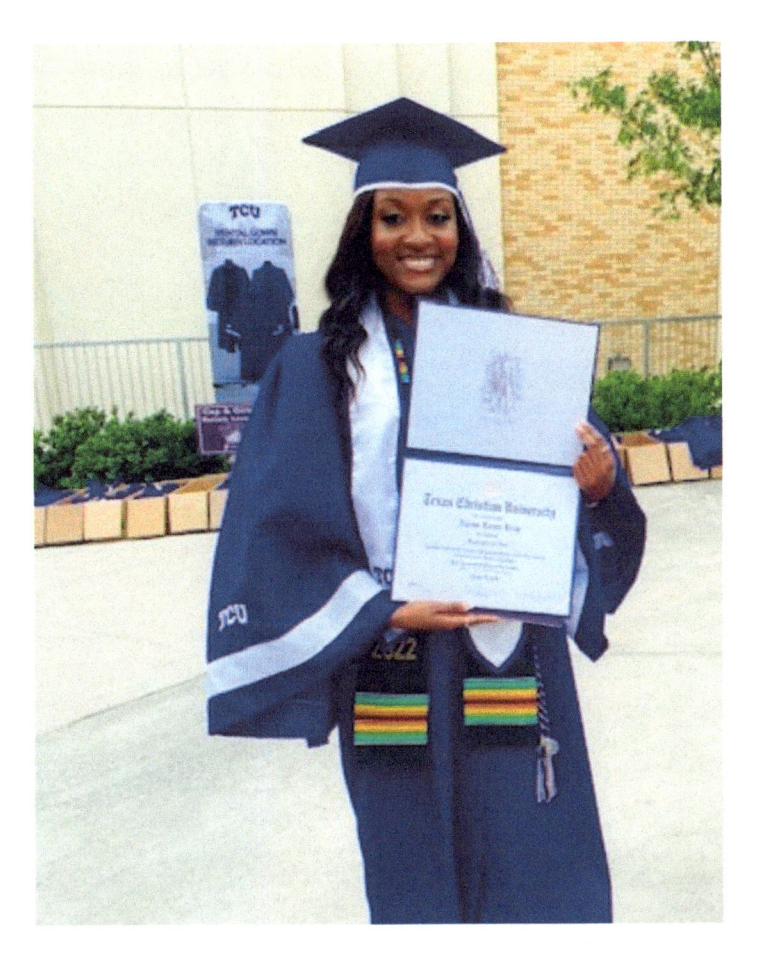

Alexis' College Graduation – Graduated on the Dean's Honor List and Cum Laude

Made in the USA
Columbia, SC
13 January 2023